AWAKEN
WELLNESS

AWAKEN WELLNESS

Taking Back the Power
to Control Your Own Health

Dr. Nicole Rothman, DC, CACCP

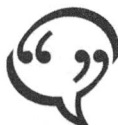

YouSpeakIt

PUBLISHING

*The Easy Way
to Get Your Book
Done Right*™

ISBN 978-1-945446-81-8

This book is dedicated to my family: my husband Troy;
Elijah and Levi, my two children; and my sweet dog, GG.
The four of you are my heart and soul.

Contents

Acknowledgments

I want to thank my husband Troy for being my person, my soulmate, my love, allowing me to be who I am, and allowing me to reach for and obtain my dreams. Your love and support are priceless.

To my children, Elijah and Levi, I thank you for understanding my schedule and my passion for what I do. I know it's not always easy having a busy mom like me, but you have been two of my greatest teachers, and I love you very much.

I want to thank my parents for their love and support and for believing in me, and my sister for her unconditional love.

Thank you to my practice members who have entrusted my team and I with their health. You pushed me to be the best doctor I can be, and I continue learning for you and from you. Thank you for the incredible Google reviews that are shared in this book to help others feel encouraged to take control of their health.

Thank you, Michelle, for introducing me to my spiritual side and for being my best friend and confidante. You were there through my entire awakening journey and still are.

Thank you to those who taught me to harness my inner power and thoughts and to appreciate and value who I am, including, but not limited to, Abraham Hicks, Deepak

Chopra, Bob Proctor, Marlo Morgan, Oprah Winfrey, Jake Ducey, Marianne Williamson, Tony Robbins, and Donny Epstein. You all helped me on my journey, and I appreciate the work you do.

Thank you to Dr. Daniel Pompa for his years of dedication to the topics of detox, fasting, and functional medicine.

Thank you to Dr. Charlie and Mindy Webb and their entire team of coaches who helped me create the practice I always wanted, made me a better doctor, and allowed me to help people in the way I always knew that I could.

Deep gratitude to my guardian angels, Sylvia, Elaine, Melissa, Michael, Ruth, Myron, Ceil, and the infinite number of other souls supporting me on this incredible journey called life.

Introduction

Awaken.

The definition of *awaken* from the Oxford Dictionary is: "to come to, come around, show signs of life, return to the land of the living, evoke, inspire, stimulate, kindle, generate, or stir."

The definition of *wellness* from the Oxford Dictionary is: ". . . the state of being in good health, especially as an actively pursued goal, an active process of becoming aware and making choices toward a healthy and fulfilling life."

This book is about awakening wellness. It gives an overview of what I teach to my practice members every day in my *Awaken Wellness* program. Health is not a destination; it's a constant, ongoing journey that one must continue throughout life. If you don't actively maintain wellness, you will move away from health again.

We all face stressors that can unravel us. Living consciously and choosing a healthy way to live is the ultimate in self-love and self-care. Making choices for the betterment of yourself and your future will impact everything: your relationships, your career, your ability to provide. It will also impact how you will spend your golden years.

The choices you make now will affect you later. There will be consequences if you don't make your health a priority.

Too often, however, we are given the idea that we have no control over our health. We are told health is predetermined by genetics, or we are treated as if we are victims under attack who can't do anything about it. Under our broken healthcare system, when health issues arise, we are told that pharmaceuticals or surgeries are the only answers.

The further we move into the broken system, the worse off most of us seem to become. Once you start on one medication, it usually leads to another and another. Many are being told that they must take the drugs for the rest of their lives. If you require drugs—even over-the-counter drugs—you are not in a state of wellness. If you have been told you need to take a medication for the rest of your life, I can promise you are not getting to the root cause of your problem.

I was a victim of this broken system for the first twenty-one years of my life. I took their pills, their allergy shots, their flu shots, sprays, steroids, antibiotics—you name it. Each year, I became more and more ill, needing more and more drugs.

It wasn't until I began to receive chiropractic care that I noticed improvements in my health. My menstrual cycle, which used to cause me severe pain, so severe I couldn't function, suddenly normalized. The pain vanished. My bowel movements became more regular. I stopped needing so many asthma medications.

At this point, I sought out different types of doctors. One had me tested for food sensitivities and told me to fast for seven days. One taught me about the gut and my body ecology and showed me how to detox.

As I explored each one of these different approaches and moved further away from conventional medicine, I became more and more healthy. I was able to eliminate or reduce my symptoms, and I needed less and less medication. My body was learning to heal itself.

I used to develop bronchitis all the time because I had severe asthma. At least three times a year, I would be on a course of antibiotics to treat bronchitis. I recall the very last time I had it. I was very sick for six weeks, during which time I refused antibiotics and medical doctors. I drank Chinese herbs, took vitamins, and got chiropractic adjustments. It took me six weeks to recover fully, but after that, I never had bronchitis again. I had allowed my body to heal itself for the first time, and I never had to do it again. My body had learned how to heal itself!

As time went on, I became more and more disenchanted with conventional medicine and conventional food. The more I healed, the more I dove into the philosophy of health and healing, the more I learned. I learned about the power our body has, the amazing, incredible restorative and regenerative properties it has. These experiences have allowed me to understand what my purpose and passion in life are:

to inspire, enlighten, educate, and empower as many people as possible to heal their own bodies so they can have the life they deserve.

This book provides you with some basic truths and gives you information necessary to begin to upgrade your health and wellness. It can help you decide what changes you would like to make and to begin planning. However, when you read this book, please realize it is a simplified overview. The rabbit hole goes deep, and there's a lot to learn. Most people need a mentor to guide them along on this process.

My sincere hope is this book empowers, encourages, and inspires you to awaken your own wellness and take control back of your own health. There is only one cure, one doctor, and it is *within you.* You need to decide if you are worth it. You are the only one who can heal your body.

P.S. Hint, hint: you are worth it.

CHAPTER ONE

Stress

Dr. Nicole Rothman Stoloff and her incredible caring team not only educate but listen, understand and care deeply and are committed to me. I remember her saying to me that weight loss will just happen as a result of your taking care of your body and supplying it with what it needs to be healthy. Your health will improve on a cellular level. I sleep better than I have in years, wake up energized, no longer have cravings, and no longer bloated. Indigestion, along with achiness, GONE! I am managing stress so much better now. So happy I have Dr. Nicole and her great support team on this journey with me. Thank you so much Dr. Nicole and staff.

~ Anita Cloutier

TYPES OF STRESS

It's not stress that kills us; it is our reaction to it.
~Hans Selye, father of stress research, MD, PhD

Stress is a critical issue to consider when it comes to wellness. Stress is capable of triggering a cascade of changes in our bodies that can ultimately cause debilitating health issues, including hormone imbalances, which can lead to inflammation and other chronic conditions down the road.

There are three different types of stress we all deal with on a regular basis. The three types of stress are *physical, emotional,* and *chemical,* and all of them can impact health. Most people won't be familiar with the concepts of physical or chemical stress; we typically only think of stress from the emotional standpoint.

We will talk about each type of stress below so you can understand how each type may affect your health, your ability to be your best, to function at your highest level, to be your healthiest, and ultimately, to have the health and the life you have always wanted to have.

Physical

Physical stress may result from accidents, like a sports injury, a car accident, or a fall. Although exercise is a healthy pursuit, your body can experience physical stress from doing too much exercise. Too little movement can also be stressful; physical stress can result from sitting too many hours a day. Electromagnetic fields (EMFs) can cause stress on our bodies; we can experience physical stress from having too many electronics around us day and night. It is important to be aware of this modern-day, invisible factor that is becoming a greater stress with every technological advancement.

Physical stresses cause chemicals to be released in our bodies that start an inflammatory response used for healing. In the short term, this is a good thing, a necessity. We need it; it's how we heal. If it becomes a chronic inflammatory issue, however, then it starts to break down the body over time, and it becomes a negative force. Inflammation is an important safeguard, and sometimes we need it, but if it continues in the long run, it can be very damaging.

Emotional

Emotional stress is the type of stress we can relate to the most. All day long, we're faced with difficulties in our lives. Driving in traffic, difficult workplace relationships, having conflict with people in our lives, having a relative who is sick, or a child who is not doing well—all these can cause emotional stress. Even just listening to the news can be stressful.

We may think this type of stress is out of our control, but many of the things we do in our regular day could be adding to our emotional stress.

For example, do you have news alerts pop up all day on your phone?

This can create enormous stress in your body. With each alert, your stress hormones spike, which can lead to anxiety, sleep issues, and even make you gain weight. You can reduce this kind of stress today simply by opting out of these notifications or deleting the apps that send you these alerts all day. They are rarely positive.

Emotional stress is under your control more than you have been led to believe. Stress is part of your life. It will never completely go away, but you can make your body more resilient and adaptable in the way it handles stress.

Other types of emotional stress we may not recognize are burdens we have been holding on to since childhood or early on in life. This kind of stress can create a pattern of thought or behavior we need to work on and break through before we can really be healthy. Looking back to the past is an important tool to learn about ourselves and heal our bodies as well. Childhood trauma can create patterns in our body that lead to dis-ease.

> *Every stress leaves an indelible scar, and the organism pays for its survival after a stressful situation by becoming a little older.*
>
> ~Hans Selye, MD, PhD

Chemical

Chemical stress is the stress people are least familiar with, but it is probably the one that is creating the biggest burden in this day and age because we aren't even aware we need to address it. We are living in a very toxic world. Toxins are in our air, our water supply, our soil, in our food. It's difficult to avoid. Medications are chemicals. Anything you put in your mouth that is not a nutrient can create stress on your body.

Any chemical substance you put on your body—even something like laundry detergent—can be creating a chemical stress you're not even aware of. You may be doing a healthy exercise program but may be doing your body damage if your pores are opening up while you're wearing a t-shirt and shorts covered in toxic laundry detergent.

This is an area we can have a ton of control over. We can minimize chemical stress in our lives when we have the right strategies in place.

I live a pretty low-chemical life, but it's hard to avoid chemical stress. One day, my husband and I were at the beach, enjoying a day out in the fresh air. We didn't anticipate we were in any chemical danger, but that day there were planes flying above dropping pesticides all over us because it was supposed to rain the next day.

This is one of the strategies our government uses to reduce mosquitoes. In an attempt to control Mother Nature, they purposely put toxins into our environment.

We sometimes don't even realize we are being exposed to pesticides falling from the sky without our knowledge. It's hard to avoid chemical stress, but it can be addressed and worked on. There are ways we can work toward eliminating or reducing it in our bodies. Regular cellular detoxification has become a necessity.

THE CHEMISTRY OF STRESS

The human body is designed to respond to stimuli in certain ways. It is part of our basic chemistry. Some simple chemical reactions have been a part of being human since we became human. We are not necessarily in the same environments we used to live in, but the same patterns of how chemicals are released in our bodies remain. The chemistry of stress is one example.

There are two key hormones involved in stress, and it is important to look at these hormones when we are trying to understand the effects of stress. However, they're often completely ignored by conventional medicine when it comes to trying to figure out what is going on with someone's health.

It's not the fault of conventional doctors; the fault lies in our system of medical education. Most medical doctors are simply not taught to seek root causes. They are mainly trained to look at symptoms and treat with medication. When the situation becomes unmanageable, often surgery is the next answer. That model of treatment of treating symptoms and ignoring the actual cause is failing miserably. Our level of health in this country proves it just doesn't work.

The Main Hormones Involved in Stress

There are two major hormones involved in the stress response. The first one is *adrenaline*. It is secreted by your adrenal glands in conditions of stress. Adrenaline typically makes your blood pump harder, gets you breathing faster, boosts your energy, increases carbohydrate metabolism, and prepares your muscles for you to run or fight. This is a fast-acting type of hormone. To understand this reaction, think about someone cutting you off when you're driving. Your heart starts beating fast, and you become panicky for a moment. However, your body recovers in less than a minute because adrenaline is quickly reabsorbed by your body.

The other hormone is *cortisol*. Adrenaline is a fat-burning hormone, whereas cortisol is a fat-storing hormone. Cortisol is typically the one that creates problems for most people. It is long acting. A study showed that after you have a tiff with your spouse or significant other, your blood pressure, blood sugar, and cortisol level can stay elevated for sixteen hours after!

In our modern age, cortisol is commonly what we're dealing with when it comes to our reactions to all types of stress, not just emotional stress. If you're eating a poor diet all the time, you can be creating cortisol as a response to that stress. If you are having a lot of physical demands that are stressful, you can cause issues with your cortisol levels. And of course, emotional stresses have an impact on stress hormones. If you have an app on your phone that sends you messages all day long telling you all the *wonderful* things that are going on in the world that day, you will be pumping this cortisol out all day long.

Cortisol is a steroid hormone. It raises your blood sugar, raises the brain's capacity to use blood sugar, and curbs other functions, such as digestion, sex drive, growth, and healing. Cortisol in the long term can impact many things, such as mood, motivation, and even your ability to feel fear or to handle life in general.

When Your Adrenals Are Out of Balance

When you have physical, emotional, and chemical stresses constantly driving the release of cortisol, your adrenals may be pumping it out all day long. This can affect the rest of your bodily systems, and can make you feel out of control with your health.

Some symptoms that can potentially result from cortisol imbalance are:

- Weight gain
- Low energy
- Difficulty sleeping
- Brain fog
- Thyroid issues

- Lowered libido
- Constipation, reflux, and other GI symptoms
- Immune suppression
- Blood sugar fluctuations
- Mood disturbances

As you can see, cortisol can have an impact on many areas of the body and on many different body functions. We will discuss each of these issues in more detail below.

Most of us complain that we are storing fat, not burning fat. This can be stimulated by the overproduction of cortisol, which is a fat-storing hormone.

Cortisol impacts energy levels. A common complaint I hear is people not having enough energy, and this can be due to a cortisol imbalance. Cortisol is responsible for your circadian rhythm, your sleep cycle. This cycle also allows you to sustain energy throughout the day. Waking up in the morning, cortisol should be high. It should slowly come down through the day so that, by nighttime, it is low enough to sleep. In some cases where the adrenals are overproducing cortisol over a long period, the adrenals can burn out. In these cases, they do not create *enough* cortisol. When the adrenals burn out, you are making enough cortisol to affect your energy levels during the day.

Your sleep cycle may be affected if your cortisol is high at night instead of being low at night. If it is not high enough in the morning, this can affect your ability to wake up feeling refreshed. It could also affect your ability to stay asleep. Sleep disturbances— waking up in the night, for instance—are another issue so many of us are facing. If you're not sleeping well, that one issue alone can create other ones, such as moodiness and energy problems leading to more of that toxic stress cycle.

Brain fog is another common symptom, and adrenal issues can create issues with brain function. We know that cortisol has a long-term impact on the brain.

Problems with the adrenal glands being out of balance can affect other organs and systems in the body. Adrenal issues can create thyroid problems because high cortisol can suppress your thyroid hormone production. Adrenal imbalances can also create sex hormone imbalances. Cortisol can suppress testosterone, for example, potentially affecting libido. In addition, adrenals that are out of balance can suppress your immune system.

Adrenal issues can also disrupt your gastrointestinal (GI) tract. Various digestive issues can result because cortisol slows digestion down. Examples of digestive issues are bloating, constipation, reflux, or diarrhea. Gastrointestinal problems can lead to all kinds of health issues, including other hormone imbalances, behavior and mood disturbances, and immune system problems.

We know cortisol raises blood sugar, so diabetes, one of the top diseases in this world right now, is another condition cortisol can impact. Looking at the levels of cortisol is an important piece of information for those who are trying to help people reverse their diabetes; yet it is often ignored.

The adrenals have an impact on our entire body. They are often overlooked because conventional medicine doesn't usually look for the cause. It only looks at the symptoms. Cortisol issues are often ignored even though we all acknowledge we have too much stress. It's important to check our adrenals to see if they are at the root of our health issues. They can cause such a drastic impact on so many different parts of the body.

Five Early Signs That Stress Is Disrupting Hormones

How do you know if stress is causing problems with your health?

There are five warning signs that stress is disrupting hormones:

- Belly fat
- Energy issues
- Brain fog
- Digestive issues
- Sleep disturbances

The one issue I probably hear about the most from people is belly fat, and this is because they want to do something about it. We are always hearing from people that they can't lose weight no matter how much they exercise or eat right. This is often because they are not addressing the underlying hormone imbalance. Stubborn belly fat is one of the signs that cortisol may be involved. Other issues, including estrogen dominance, thyroid deficiencies, and insulin resistance, could lead to weight gain.

The other four early warning signs—energy issues, brain fog or mental sluggishness, digestive issues, and sleep disturbances—are often seen as normal signs of aging, so we rarely pay attention to them.

Because we are taught that these are normal signs of aging, nobody is telling us there might be a problem. Nobody is telling us it's not normal to wake up at three o'clock in the morning. People think it's because they are fifty years old, and it's normal. They think that brain fog and lowered energy are to be expected once you get to a certain age.

However, these five warning signs may mean you already have a problem.

It is not normal to wake up in the middle of the night. You should be sleeping through the night. It's not normal to have brain fog and low energy. Unpleasant GI symptoms are not normal. We need to look at those as early as possible before we get into a bigger health crisis down the road.

It's very rare that I see people come in who don't have issues with cortisol if they are experiencing issues with energy or sleep. If cortisol is too high or low during the day, the circadian rhythms of the body are affected.

Abnormal cortisol levels can have a debilitating effect on health and quality of life. Donna, one of my practice members, came to me with severe anxiety. She was unable to drive on the highway. We found out that her cortisol was extremely low, and the low cortisol was creating anxiety for her.

We were able to help her with:

1. Lifestyle changes
2. Detoxification
3. Nutrition
4. Nutraceuticals to support her adrenals (to balance her cortisol)
5. Chiropractic care to reduce stress on her nervous system

Now, she functions normally without anxiety interfering in her life. Her blood pressure has normalized. She has been able to go on living life the way she should be able to, including driving her car wherever she wants to go. Donna followed the *Awaken Wellness* blueprint and took back control of her health.

THE KEYS TO REDUCING STRESS

We all hear about ways to reduce stress: yoga, meditation, deep breathing.

Is this what we should be doing?

It's important we understand a few things in order to know how we can really, truly be reducing stress in our lives.

The Truth

Here's the deal. The truth is you're being lied to when it comes to health and wellness.

Sickness is a multi-billion-dollar industry based on you being sick. The pharmaceutical and the insurance industries make more money the sicker you are. Most of the advice we're getting out there—which we see in every other commercial on TV—tells us to go ask our doctor for the next best chemical for our illness.

These chemicals are not going to fix you or your life. They are not going to heal you or get to the root cause of what is going on with you. When we talk about stress, we need to look at all types of stress—physical, chemical, and emotional. We can't just *om* our way to health. It doesn't work like that. It helps, but it's only one piece of the solution.

We must understand this is a big business. It's quite obvious the treatment-oriented system is failing. Just look at the numbers. All the chronic degenerative diseases we see so many suffer from continue to rise in numbers even though we are spending billions on medical treatments. This all leads to just as much disease, if not more, than before. Heart disease, diabetes, cancer, autoimmune, obesity—the numbers keep climbing.

Conventional treatment means being offered either medicine or surgery to address symptoms. If we want to heal our bodies, regain our health, and turn our lives around, we're going to have to do this on an individual level by stepping outside the conventional medicine box of prescribing, diagnosis, and treatment. We must find the *root cause*.

Physical, emotional, and chemical stressors are at the root of health issues, and they are not being addressed properly. You must dig down to the root cause to take back control of your health and life.

We're in Control of Our Health

We are being told, repeatedly, that we're not in control of our health—or our lives, for that matter. We are told we should blame external factors, like stress, the economy, our genes, our boss, or the other people around us. We are told we're not in control of our health; we are victims of circumstance.

This is not the truth. You do have control, and it's time to take responsibility for your health—and for your life, if it's not how you want it to be. If you don't take responsibility, there will be consequences. Awaken wellness.

If you don't pay your taxes, you will owe a debt to the IRS. In the same way, if you don't take responsibility for your health and invest time, energy, and money into it, you will owe a debt that you will eventually have to pay.

You might say that some health problems are the result of accidents no one has control over. Yes, a physical injury can sometimes result from a random event you couldn't have avoided—although I do believe we attract what happens to us. However, you do have the ability to minimize the effects of even this kind of an accident.

For example, how about getting your body into a more resilient and flexible state so that if you are injured, you can handle it better?

It's like being a piece of spaghetti. If you are an uncooked piece of spaghetti, I can snap you right in half because if you are not flexible. However, if I cook you and throw you against the wall, you're not going to fall apart. You will be less likely to be injured because you're much more resilient. We have the ability to improve our bodies; we can make them more flexible and resilient.

We can make our nervous systems stronger to remove any interference. Meditating and doing abdominal breathing exercises help us get our nervous systems into a healthier state. Chiropractic care helps many people by reducing interference and stress in the nervous system and making it more adaptable. We are in control of our nervous system health.

What about genetics? Can't we blame our health problems on our genes?

It's become commonplace for people to blame everything on genetics. Blaming your health issues on genetics means you have no option, no way out, no choice. However, we know for a fact that genes are only a small percentage, under 5 percent, directly related to health conditions. Epigenetic research tells us it's our lifestyle and environment that determine whether a gene expresses itself or not.

Lifestyle trumps genetics any day. It is your lifestyle that determines how much stress you put on your body, and you are in control of your lifestyle.

Know that there is only one person who can get you well, who can help you, who can take charge: *you.* You're the only person who can turn your health around. It's a choice for you to make. Make the decision to take control.

Your power has been taken from you in the past. Take it back. Only you can Awaken Wellness for yourself.

Addressing Stress

Emotional stress isn't the only kind of stress we need to monitor. In order to be healthy, we have to address all types of stress.

If you're not exercising or moving your body enough, you need to address that. If you are sitting all day, especially if in a poor position, you need to make some changes. You can stand up and take a walk around the building; you can make ergonomic changes to make that space better for your body. You can set an alarm on your phone to remind yourself to get up and move every thirty or forty minutes so you are not sitting there for hours. You can stretch, go on a lunch break, and go on a brisk walk to get the blood moving. There are ways to address stress. We are in control.

Mindset is critical, and we'll be talking about it more later in the book. Having a positive mindset is necessary for addressing stress, for being able to let things slide off you, to recognize that life is good, and to have gratitude.

We must take control over chemical stress. We're the ones who decide what chemicals surround our bodies and homes. You decide what to put in your body, what to put on your body, what to clean your home with, what to clean your clothing with. You decide if you're going to spray perfume on your body or use natural essential oils instead. These are all decisions we make every single day, although many of us are not even aware that there is a decision to make.

We need to become empowered in this area. It is an area we are poorly educated in. We trust that our government is protecting us, and that industries are acting according to health standards. The truth is the Environmental Working Group has found in the cord blood of infants that our babies are being exposed to almost three hundred chemicals before they are even born.[1]

1"Body Burden: Pollution in Newborns," Environmental Working

We need to start making different choices. We must become knowledgeable, empowered, and educated, particularly in the area of chemical stress, because we are constantly being exposed to things we're not even aware of. Awareness is what is going to change our health and change the future for our children's health as well. Awaken Wellness for the future.

Awareness must then be followed by action. Knowledge is powerful, but only if you apply it.

> *Choosing Rothman Health Solutions was the best decision I could have made for my health! I have struggled for 25+ years with declining health and I'm only forty years old. I've tried multiple diets, [a] nutritionist, personal trainers, and even consulted and approved [for] bariatric surgery. I've seen many doctors/specialist[s] and never any answers. I just kept getting more labels and medications. A few of my symptoms included fatigue, depression, high blood pressure, insulin resistance, migraines, hair loss, facial hair growth, adrenal fatigue, hypothyroidism, brain fog, no restful sleep, depression, and the list continued . . . In six months with Dr. Rothman, many of the above symptoms are gone. I have a regular sleep schedule and wake up restful, total weight loss of forty-five pounds, have energy to do things instead of sleeping all day, no migraines, no depression, good*

Group, (July 14, 2005), www.ewg.org/research/body-burden-pollution-newborns

blood pressure, facial hair has declined, no brain fog or depression. I am now in control of my health because of the education I received from Rothman Health Solutions. I still have some work to do, but I learned what works for me! There is no standard to fit everyone, but with the proper testing and education, everyone can be in charge of their own health!

~ Amber Lawson Griggs

CHAPTER TWO

True Detoxification

TOXINS: THE THREE MAIN CULPRITS

We must address the toxic burden we have in this world. We have toxins in our food, in our air, in our soil. They are all around us, indoors as well as outdoors. In fact, the air inside the home is typically way more toxic than outside the home. It's a huge issue. The toxic burden that we're facing is one of the most difficult health challenges to overcome.

There are many different toxins. In this section, we'll talk about the three main types of toxins that may be holding you back from achieving the health you should have.

These three main culprits are:

- Heavy metals
- Molds
- Hidden infections

Heavy Metals

Heavy metals have been an ongoing health issue for many generations. The three main toxic heavy metals we're dealing with are mercury, aluminum, and lead.

Mercury

Mercury accumulation often comes from amalgam fillings, which are not safe for our bodies. We know that mercury is the most neurotoxic substance on the planet. It is not safe to have it in our teeth. The mercury vapors constantly coming off these fillings may impact the brain, particularly the hypothalamus. Metal fillings, however, continue to be used because they last a long time. I have no idea who came up with the genius idea to put this metal in our mouths, but it's time to get them out and admit it was not a smart move.

Having these amalgams in your mouth—even if they are tiny pieces—will hold you back from having your best health. We are also exposed to mercury in some vaccines, by consuming fish, and with exposure to pesticides. Mercury tends to make its way to the brain quickly and accumulates there.

Aluminum

People cook in aluminum cookware. There is aluminum in antiperspirant deodorant. We are wrapping and cooking our food in aluminum foil. Aluminum is now used in most vaccines, to replace mercury, but aluminum is just as toxic in its own way. Aluminum also has an affinity for the brain tissues and has been linked to Alzheimer's as far back as the 1970s by Dr. Hugh Fudenberg.[2]

Lead

Our generation is not exposed the same way to lead as previous generations who were exposed to paint, crystal, and even gasoline. These days lead can be in our water from pipes, soil, pottery, and cosmetics, lipsticks being the highest exposure. Lead that enters our bodies is usually stored in our bones. When we lose bone density for any reason, lead is released into the body. This also happens during pregnancy to the mother as she grows the fetus in her womb. These metals go deep into the tissues. Until we get them out of the body and the brain, we can never fully get our health back.

Molds

Many of us are exposed to mold without even knowing it. We can be living in a building that has had water damage, where mold is hidden away in places where you can't see it. This happened in my house. There was a leak from the air conditioning handler in our garage, and it was blowing mold spores throughout our entire house without our knowledge.

2 Fudenberg, Hugh. "Hazards of Vaccines 1, 2." *International Journal of Clinical Investigation.* 2000 and 2004.

Down in Florida where I live, everybody is exposed to mold on a regular basis just by being outside. Think about all the storms and hurricanes we have had over the years. We live in a very humid environment, so it's hard to avoid exposure. Mold may accumulate in older homes and in buildings where people work and shop. Toxic algae can be problematic as well.

When your immune system is unable to handle mold, it can even accumulate inside your body. This causes massive problems, particularly with chronic inflammatory issues such as *chronic inflammatory response syndrome* (CIRS) and can even lead to diseases, such as Alzheimer's.

The biggest problem with molds is the toxins they may release. The toxins themselves are what will cause the biggest health issues. Many of us don't have the ability to detox these out of our bodies; our immune systems can't handle them well. Many people don't realize this is causing their health issues.

Hidden Infections

Hidden infections are infections in your body that don't have typical symptoms like fever, pain, and swelling. They are often difficult to diagnose. These kinds of hidden infections are examples of what I call *upstream issues,* which we will be talking more about in the next section. To turn someone's health around, we often have to uncover and address hidden infections to find the root cause of the problem.

Hidden infections can come in many forms, including:

- Fungal infections
- Bacterial infections
- Viral infections
- Parasites

A hidden fungal infection may result from the overgrowth of a yeast organism like *candida*. For example, you can have a candida overgrowth in your gut that can cause health issues. In some cases, the candida can also leave your gut for other locations, especially if gut inflammation causes you to have a condition called *leaky gut*—which we'll talk more about later in the book. Because of steroids, antibiotics, hormone replacement, and birth control pills, candida infections are very common. These drugs kill the good gut bugs and leave candida to overpopulate. As an additional complication, you can't have a candida infection without having some heavy metal toxicity. These organisms live off heavy metals.

A hidden bacterial infection may result from overgrowth of bacteria. For example, certain opportunistic bacteria may multiply in your colon or small intestine, causing health problems. There are also numerous viral infections you may unknowingly pick up. Some well-known hidden viral infections are Epstein-Barr virus, human papilloma virus (HPV), herpes, and varicella virus. These viruses can play a role influencing in our long-term health.

Some parasites may cause hidden infections. Because we live in America and think our country is so clean, many people don't realize that we are exposed to parasites too. Parasitic infections are also often associated with heavy metal toxicity.

Infections may be hiding in areas of the body where we don't expect to find them. For example, we may see infections in dental work, where you have an implant in your mouth. A low-lying infection can develop around these implants.

You can develop infections where you've had a tooth pulled. If the bone doesn't close up all the way, this could leave a little cave where it's dark and warm so viruses or bacteria—like the Lyme bacterium, for instance—can easily live and breed. These *cavitations,* as we call them, can create serious health problems for people, and you may not even know they're there. You may not know when an infection develops in these hidden places if you don't have typical symptoms like pain, inflammation, or fever.

Another area where a hidden infection might reside is in root canals. The only time we ever leave a dead body part in the body is when we save a tooth and kill the nerve, which is its life source, and leave the dead tooth in the body. In these cases, a hidden infection may occur around the root. A good way we can check the teeth for these types of infections is with a special 3D cone beam X-ray, with the diagnostic software to read it properly.

A biofilm, which is a layer of microbes lining a surface, can develop around implanted material, whether it is a hip replacement or a screw in a bone, and this may result in infections that can be there for long periods without us ever knowing it. These underlying, long-term, hidden, chronic infections may create an inflammatory response in the body. As we've already discussed, inflammation is a natural immune response, but ultimately, it can lead to many different types of health issues down the road.

Heavy metals, molds, and hidden infections must all be eliminated when trying to regain health. As we've seen, these culprits may be related to each other, which makes their assessment even more complicated. We have to address each issue, as well as address their relationships with each other.

WHAT DOES A REAL DETOX LOOK LIKE?

When it comes to detoxification, there is a lot of confusion. A real detox looks very different from what most people might think. We associate the word with a variety of activities that involve just a few weeks of misery. Maybe we lose a little bit of weight; maybe we'll have to sit on the toilet often in an effort to clean out our bowels; maybe we're not able to leave the house for these weeks. However, a real detox must go deeper to truly Awaken Wellness.

We can't just clean up the colon to return to health. Colon cleanses will never get us completely well. The three major toxins we discussed in the last section are not typically addressed in your everyday, multilevel-marketed juice-fast program, or another quick-fix colon cleanse. We have to go much deeper than that. In order to go deeper, you have to use specific strategies and formulas; you really have to hit the problem head-on. A real detox has to heal at a cellular level.

Start Downstream and Work Our Way Upstream

The colon, liver, and kidneys are vital for detoxifying and eliminating, and they are what we call the *downstream* organs. We will begin with improving the functioning of these downstream organs when we are trying to improve body health. However, that isn't enough. We also need to move *upstream* to address other parts of the body. We need to take care of our health at a cellular level.

We need to repair the cells of the body. Our cell membranes are damaged and inflamed by exposure to stress and toxins. When these membranes are inflamed, the good things, like hormones and nutrients, can't get into the cells, and the bad things can't get out. Accumulated toxins from the environment and from your own cellular waste build up inside your cells.

Your body uses foods as fuel for energy. You know that when your car uses fuel for energy, it leaves waste behind. It's the same in your cells. We produce waste during our metabolic activities, and that waste needs to be removed or it will become toxic.

We start our detox with the gut and the lower downstream organs. Once those are healthier and can process toxins better, we go deeper and clean up the body. This deep cleansing is relatively easy when we have already improved the health of the liver, kidneys, and digestive tract. When these organs are able to process wastes more easily and move them out of the body faster, we can go deeper into the cells to get rid of the toxicity in the cells.

But we still need to go even further upstream. The brain is next. We can't work on detoxing the brain until the body and the downstream organs are ready to remove the toxins that accumulate in the brain over the course of life. Many of these toxins love fat. Your brain is made up of 80 percent fat, so toxins have an affinity for the brain, and they are easily stored there.

For truly effective detoxing, we have to go in steps, in layers. We can't move on to the next phase until one phase is done.

Time and Testing

While you are working on detoxifying, as time passes, it is natural to wonder:

Am I progressing at all?

How well am I doing with this detox?

It's important that we use a gauge to check the progress of a detox, but you need to understand that everybody is different. We all want to feel like we're making progress, but not everybody moves forward at the same rate. When it comes to timing, everybody is different.

We will use regular testing to determine how far you've come, how well your body is eliminating toxins, and if you need to continue using the detoxification strategies we've taught you.

We use these three tests to assess the progress of a detox:

- Meta-oxy urine test
- Visual contrast sensitivity test
- Symptom questionnaire

The *meta-oxy urine test* looks for a substance called malondialdehyde. It is a marker for oxidative stress and cell membrane inflammation and damage. The higher the amount of cell membrane inflammation, damage, and oxidative stress you have, the more malondialdehyde will be in your urine. This goes on a scale of zero to seven. We want you close to zero. Zero, one, or two are passing. Anything higher than that means we have to continue to detox.

The *visual contrast sensitivity test* was created by Dr. Ritchie Shoemaker. He is one of the top mold doctors in our country and is known for his strategies to help people with mold toxicity. We use the visual contrast sensitivity test to determine what different types of toxins—biotoxins, neurotoxins, general toxicity, even vitamin deficiency—you have.

Our questionnaire enables us to see how toxins are affecting your symptoms. Email me at drnicole@drnicole.com, and I will email you a free NTQ to determine your toxicity levels and analysis.

We want you to be able to pass all three tests. Dr. Dan Pompa, whom I have to thank for figuring out the best detox protocols, taught me that even after you pass all three of these tests, you should continue to detox for six months— that's how toxic we are!

It definitely takes time. Most people can't detox in just a few months because they have so much toxicity. At a minimum, you will want to do three months of detoxing. At that time, we will retest you. Then we will talk about strategies such as dealing with mold in the home, metals in your mouth, and previous dental work that may need to be checked.

We want you to get all the way through the detoxification process. That is why we use the testing. Some people take a few months, but most people take longer than that, possibly even over a year, to fully detox the body.

Binders to Remove Toxins

Binders play an important role in the detoxification process. They bind to toxins like heavy metals and carry them out of the body. The choice of binder is important. A weak binder may successfully attach to a targeted metal, but if the bond is too weak to carry them completely out of the body, the metal ends up recirculating back in. Some examples of weak binders are chlorella and cilantro.

We can get the body to release toxins, to release heavy metals, and to release different biotoxins like mold and yeast, but we need strong binders to aid this process. If the toxins circulate back into the system, *autointoxication* occurs when they settle in somewhere else. This creates a new problem. Using weak binders isn't a good strategy in the long run.

To resolve underlying issues and maintain good health, we have to use good strong binders specifically designed to help move these toxins out of the body. Some need to be small enough to cross through the blood/brain barrier. Some we want to cross into the cells to remove toxins. However, we don't want them all going inside the cell. We want some to stay outside the cell. We want to keep the binders floating around so if anything escapes, they are ready to catch it. We call these binders blood cleansers. We use an amazing product called *Cytodetox™* for this purpose. It is a cleaned clinoptilolyte, a very specialized cage to capture toxins and hold them.

We also want to set up what I think of as a *catcher's* mitt in your gut. Let me explain. During the process of removing toxins, your body creates a toxic bile complex in your gut. That bile is likely to get reused; it recirculates back into your system. Your body tends to try to conserve energy and tries to avoid having to make new things. It recycles, and one of the things it recycles is bile. Therefore, we need to detach those toxins from the bile before it leaves the gut and circulates back in. That's why we need a strong binder—a catcher's mitt—in the gut, to make sure that something is breaking that bile complex down and carrying it out of the body. We use *Bind™* from Systemic Formulas to achieve this.

The binders we use are strong and specifically designed to bind to biotoxins and remove them. Without proper binders, it would be impossible to rid the body of these havoc-wreaking toxins. When it comes to detoxing, the goal is to get these toxins out of your body, out of your cells, out of your brain, and into the toilet.

THE FIVE RS: FIVE REQUIREMENTS OF DETOXIFICATION

It is easy to find advice about detoxing from doctors, health coaches, and online experts. You will hear stories from people who feel like they've helped themselves by detoxing on their own. They typically give their bodies more nutrients and better supplements and eat a less inflammatory diet. As a result, they might genuinely feel better. However, that doesn't mean they've detoxed properly, completely, or safely.

In this section, we will describe the safe and thorough process we use to detoxify. We follow a series of steps called the *Five Rs.*

The *Five Rs* are also known as the *Five Requirements of Detoxification* because this is what is absolutely required to get your health back. We have to fix the cell in order to get you well, and the *Five Rs* will take you through that process. We will discuss each step below.

The *Five Rs* are:

- *R1* Remove the source
- *R2* Regenerate the cell membrane
- *R3* Restore cellular energy
- *R4* Reduce cellular inflammation
- *R5* Reestablish methylation

R1—Remove the Source

Removing the source of the toxicity can be accomplished in a few ways. We recommend anyone who has mercury amalgams in their mouth have them removed. If you have breast implants, they could also be causing a problem. Breast implants contain forty neurotoxins in the shell alone, so some people may need to remove their implants. We ask you to look at your home and surroundings for sources of toxicity. If there is water damage in your home, for instance, you should remediate the water damage and remove any mold.

These are all examples of removing superficial sources of toxicity. However, the key to the *Five Rs* is to focus on the cellular level. When toxins have accumulated in your cells over the years, we need to remove them. These sources cause body-wide damage and must be dealt with. We have special formulas and binders to remove the toxins from your cells and safely usher them out of your body using our protocols.

R2—Regenerate the Cell Membrane

We mentioned earlier that cell membrane damage and inflammation are some of the biggest issues when it comes to healing your body. If the cell membrane is inflamed, the toxins can't get out and the nutrients can't go in. The nutrients should flow easily into the cell. The toxins and free radicals should be easily shuttled out. If the membrane is inflamed, this cannot happen, and you will become more and more toxic.

This inflammation compromises the ability of the cell to function properly. Hormones become blocked, and then the cell can't *hear* the hormone messages. We must fix the cell membrane in order to correct this situation. We raise the levels of *glutathione,* your body's primary antioxidant, inside the cell, and we use special fats to assist in the repair process because your cell membrane is made of fat.

It's important to provide the body with the right dietary fats. Some fats, including some vegetable oils that people eat, attach to the phospholipid cell membrane and drive inflammation. Phospholipids are a combination of fats and phosphate groups that make up the membrane of every cell. Vegetable oils destroy a healthy cell membrane because they can attach to the cell as if they were a proper fat. Many people think simply taking fish oil is adequate, but you need a proper balance of omegas to heal the cell.

R3—Restore Cellular Energy

We have been talking about the outer membrane of the cell so far. There are also inner membranes, such as those of the powerhouse of the cell, the mitochondria. The mitochondrial membranes may also become inflamed. Mitochondria produce ATP, which you may have heard of. That is the energy unit of the cell. If your mitochondria cannot produce ATP properly, or the ATP cannot get into the cell properly because of the mitochondrial membrane inflammation, then you are not going to have enough fuel to get through the day.

There are interesting studies that show that athletes have more mitochondria and sick people have fewer.[3], [4]We need to create more mitochondria in the cell so we can get the body going. We need to restore these fuel regenerators. That will make a huge change for people.

3 University of Southern Denmark Faculty of Health Sciences. "New research on the muscles of elite athletes: When quality is better than quality." *Science Daily.* 02 November 2016. sciencedaily.com/releases/2016/11/161102132208.htm

4 Nunnari, Jodi and Anu Suomalainen. "Mitochondria: In Sickness and in Health." *Cell.* 16 March 2012. doi.org/10.1016/j.cell.2012.02.035

R4—Reduce Cellular Inflammation

Reducing cellular inflammation is a key component of reducing chronic degenerative conditions we see today, even cancer. Where cell membranes, particularly the mitochondrial membrane, are inflamed, we need antioxidants. The right combination of antioxidants will help to regulate inflammation.

We also need to work on how we become inflamed in the first place. Toxins can be playing a role. The type of food someone is eating will definitely play a role in this as well. We want to bring about an overall reduction in inflammation in the whole body, and this can't be accomplished by just taking supplements. However, we do find that certain antioxidants and nutrients are beneficial in achieving a reduction in cellular inflammation.

R5—Reestablish Methylation

Methylation refers to the addition of methyl groups to DNA molecules. This process is a pathway that our body uses to detoxify itself.

Our body needs these methyl groups to turn stress hormones on and off. Often, these groups become depleted because the body stays in a stressful state all the time. Some people have problems in their genes with methyl groups. They come in short supply, or they are nonexistent.

Methyl groups play a key role in detoxification and protecting your DNA, as well as a role in hormone metabolism and epigenetic mechanisms. We know we can use the *Five Rs* to turn off bad genes. These methyl groups help us to remove toxic hormones such as estrogen, but if there is too much stress, too many toxins, we can develop hormone issues. We know people under very high stress will have that problem, and it has become common.

Maintaining Your Health After the Five Rs

Think of your body as a bucket. Imagine the toxins that surround you in your daily life are the liquids that slowly fill that bucket. Eventually, that bucket can overflow. Applying the *Five Rs* principles as a road map to fix the cell, we must open and support critical detoxification pathways and use true binders to remove the toxins from the cell. This is the true path to real detoxification.

Once we reestablish these methylation pathways and our bodies are cleaned up, we also want to make sure we maintain these pathways. Stresses are going to continue. Life is going to continue. We must continue to maintain these pathways.

This means keeping inflammation down, making sure cellular energy is kept up, making sure that we continue healing the cell membrane and keep it healed, and staying consciously aware of our lifestyles so we can keep the source of these toxins down. This is the way we Awaken Wellness, take the power back and be in control of our health.

I'm so grateful that I finally found a doctor who not only actually knows what's wrong with my health, but cares about me and my health. She has the program to help fix me, and I have never felt better in my entire life! Everyone in the office is amazing! I feel like I have another family!

~ Miss Brandy

CHAPTER THREE

Healing the Gut

NOURISHING THE GUT

We're finally realizing that healing the gut is one of the main paths to healing the entire body. Your digestive tract is designed to break down food and absorb nutrients, but in addition, it has an impact on your hormones, your weight, your emotional state, and your immune system. In fact, 80 percent of the immune system lies around the colon area of the body. Issues with digestive tract health can result in many additional health problems.

The gut is a very long tube designed to digest and assimilate nutrients, and to eliminate toxins and wastes. It is very long because it takes a good amount of time and energy to do this right. It's important to understand that the food you put into your body has a substantial impact on the digestive tube that runs from your mouth all the way to the other end. Most of us look at it as just a mechanical tube, but the health of the gut can easily impact the health of the rest of our body.

Your *gut microbiome*—the collection of beneficial microbes that live in your gut—is of great importance. There are approximately one hundred trillion bacteria in and on our body, the majority of which are in our gut. Feeding the microbiome, as well as feeding our body properly, is going to have a tremendous impact on our overall health.

Inflammation, medications, stress, unhealthy foods, infections, toxins, and heavy metals can all contribute to a condition that has become more common than not—*leaky gut*. When you have this condition, it means that your intestinal barrier is no longer a good barrier. The tight junctions along the intestinal wall weaken and open, allowing food particles, bacteria, candida, etc., to leak out.

Leaky gut is why we are seeing the development of food sensitivities. When your body looks at a food and thinks of it as a foreign invader, it launches an immune response, which creates an inflammatory response, which is part of how you get sick. Inflammation is one of the roots of all disease.

How does the gut get damaged enough to become a leaky gut in the first place?

The first factor is stress. You are probably aware that stress and mood have an impact on your gastrointestinal system. Many report digestive trouble in times of stress. It can even happen when you're just nervous or excited about something. However, when we're talking about stress, this doesn't only mean the emotional kind. Physical stress or chemical stress can be damaging to the gut as well. It's important we address all stress in order to prevent and reverse damage of the gut.

Medications damage our microbiome. We know that antibiotics are one of the worst culprits out there because they can kill many of your good bacteria, which play a critical role in your immune system. Those good bacteria keep the bad bacteria and other opportunistic organisms at bay. When we wipe out the good guys, the bad guys can overgrow.

Steroids, cortisol, and hormones, like birth control pills, can also harm our gut integrity. NSAIDS, such as aspirin, ibuprofen, or naprosyn are also destructive to your gut flora. Think about the birth control pill. We have generations of women who have been taking hormones for many years. Now, we seem to have an epidemic of people who have a difficult time getting pregnant. Gut health issues can lead to hormone imbalances. Our gut health has been drastically impacted by the birth control pill.

Foods that contain GMOs, sugars, alcohol, artificial sweeteners, and human-made fats can impact your gut health. Environmental toxins, found in your home or your yard or from cleaning products and cosmetic products, can also cause gut issues.

These damaging foods, medications, infections, and toxins, combined with stress, can result in a leaky gut. Healing this leaky gut—as well as healing the gut itself—is an absolute pillar of healing the body. It must happen. It's non-negotiable.

You will be spinning your wheels if you are trying to knock out a candida infection without trying to heal the gut, or if you are trying to lose weight without trying to heal the gut. The gut is the source of many of our health issues.

The Gut-Damaging Foods

Any food that is not a real food can damage the gut. For example, genetically modified foods, which are not made by nature, can damage the digestive tract. They are altered by humans and may be loaded with *glyphosate*. Only foods labeled organic are guaranteed to be free of this chemical. Glyphosate has already been found to cause inflammation, and glysophate use has been associated with an increased risk of cancer. We know GMOs create a difference in our gut microbiome and have a negative impact on our overall health and wellness. Everybody is different, but we know that choosing foods in their most natural state is healthier for us all.

Gluten has become well-known as an inflammatory food. It can actually tear the gut lining when you eat it. Our body has an amazing capacity to heal, but eventually, if it tears enough times, it may not heal.

Sugar and artificial sweeteners have a detrimental effect because sugar can feed bad bugs that are in the gut. Artificial sweeteners like Splenda are damaging our microbiome by killing off good bacteria.

Other foods bad for our gut health are bad fats such as vegetable oils, oils processed with heat, and hydrogenated oils. These oils create more inflammation.

Processed foods, farmed fish, conventional meat, poultry, and dairy can be detrimental. Even vegetables like eggplant and tomatoes—the nightshade vegetables—can be damaging for some.

Our water supply could also be impacting us. Water is recycled; chlorine, fluoride, and other toxins are being dumped into our water supply. Medications and hormones that we are excreting, as well as other environmental toxins, are added into the water as it is recycled. Our water supply could be damaging our gut as well.

The Gut-Healing Foods

There are some Awaken Wellness foods that can help to heal the gut, and it's a good idea to consume a variety of these foods. We want to try to bring diversity to the gut flora. The more good stuff we pass through the gut the healthier it will be.

Here are just a few options:

- Bone broth
- Organ meats
- Fermented foods
- Kefir, raw dairy, or kefir water
- Prebiotic foods

- Organic vegetables
- Non-inflammatory fats and oils

One of my favorites of the gut-healing foods is bone broth. Bone broth is basically a broth made with healthy bones— beef bones, bison bones, lamb bones, chicken, turkey, and fish—from grass-fed or pastured, organic animals. This broth is loaded with nutrients like glutamine, proline, glycine, collagen, minerals, and arginine, which are all especially important when it comes to healing that intestinal barrier and creating tight junctions in the gut.

Organ foods are nutrient dense and can provide special benefits. For example, consuming liver from a healthy animal can help us repair our liver. Having a healthy liver is vitally important to healthy detoxification, balanced hormones, digestion, and blood sugar.

Fermented foods are highly beneficial and healing to our gut. The fermentation of veggies, like the cooking of bone broth, is an old, traditional food preparation, dating far back to our early ancestors. Prior to refrigeration, fermented vegetables were extremely common, and they are still easy to find. Fermented veggies are loaded with beneficial probiotics. Kimchi and sauerkraut, the versions that are alive and not processed, are beneficial. You can ferment all different types of vegetables.

Kefir is another option. You don't want to use conventional dairy. If you are drinking dairy kefir, you want to make sure your milk is raw, from grass-fed cows, and organic. You can also have something like coconut milk kefir, which is my favorite. Kefir strains are also used to ferment waters. Sometimes there is fruit added to flavor it but be careful of consuming too much sugar in store-bought versions.

We also have *prebiotic* foods to heal the gut. These are certain foods that feed the microbiome. Try asparagus, garlic, onion, chicory root, jicama, artichoke, and dandelions. We know that when your diet is higher in vegetables, this changes your whole microbiome. You will ingest different bacteria that are sending different messages; we want them to send healthy messages to create more health.

We know your gut can affect your senses, such as how you taste foods. I often hear my practice members say that when they started eating healthier, their taste buds changed. Well, you are changing your whole body. You are changing your microbiome. You are changing your gut with these healthy foods, and as a result, you might experience differences in flavor, texture, and even sight or sound.

We also want to be giving the gut healthy fats, like avocados, coconut oil, cold-pressed, organic olive oil, raw and even soaked and sprouted seeds and nuts. These are healthy fats for most people. Peanuts and cashews for some may be the exception; they can be inflammatory. Most of the other nuts and seeds are tolerable. These are some of the very best foods. Coconut oil is one of my favorites because it has caprylic acid, which is beneficial for the gut and can be helpful with candida overgrowth.

Some supplements can also be helpful for healing the gut. We will discuss supplements later in this book.

Testing Your Food Sensitivities

We have found that food sensitivities can be a vitally important issue for inflammatory conditions. When you are trying to turn your health around, you should determine if you are sensitive to any particular foods.

Now, you can do the standard dietary elimination diet, where you eliminate the standard inflammatory foods, and slowly add them back one by one to see how you react. We recommend doing this because it's important you listen to your body. How your body responds always takes priority over any test. We have been taught to ignore our bodies instead of listening to the messages they send us. It's amazing how quickly someone feels better just from eliminating sugar alone!

These elimination foods are:

- Sugar
- Artificial sweeteners
- Juice
- Dairy
- Soy

- Eggs
- Shellfish
- Tomatoes
- Peanuts
- Grains
- Gluten

As we've discussed, you eliminate these foods and then add them back one at a time, recording any changes in the way you feel. Awareness develops from this process.

However, when it comes to delayed food sensitivity, sometimes it's difficult to determine if a food you're eating today is affecting you when you don't notice anything until three days later. We like to test for foods that may have these delayed reactions. This means determining if your body is creating an inflammatory response to a food you ate four days ago.

The IgG part of your immune system is responsible for delayed food sensitivity. When you are tested for allergies, you are typically tested for IgE, which is an immediate response. An IgG reaction is an all-out immune launch where the body thinks a food is attacking it much like a bacteria or virus. So, an inflammatory response occurs and can last for up to four days.

The FIT Test employs unique methods that detect both IgG antibodies and complement antigen together to determine the reactivity of each sample against a wide variety of food antigens. These methods yield more complete profiles of the various foods that may cause food sensitivities.

To accomplish this, I use a food test that not only measures IgG, but also what we call a complement. There are a few different tests. There is one test that we use where twenty-two of the top foods show up the most, and there are labs, called FIT 22, that test up to 300 different types of food. Over the years, we have found that it is very rare to not find any sensitivities. Likely, this result is because so many people have gut issues that lead to immune system disruptions.

Identifying foods that cause inflammation can make all the difference in the world to your healing. The more inflammation you have, the harder it is to overcome whatever other health challenges you're dealing with. I find addressing food sensitivities to be a necessary component to helping our practice members improve their health.

KILLING OFF THE BAD BUGS

When we talk about killing, we need to understand that there is more to gut health, and more to our health in general, than just wiping out populations of bad bugs. That is what antibiotics attempt to do, and it hasn't been working.

There is a reason why a body has an overgrowth of organisms like candida, bacteria, or parasites. Just killing off those bad bugs and infections is not going to move you all the way to good health. Those bugs are there because their food supply is there and because they can find what they need to survive. The bugs live and multiply because your immune system isn't strong enough to fight them off. If we really want to address this as a systemic and whole-body issue, we need to address the cause of the biotoxin overgrowth.

Therefore, we must work on killing them off while we eliminate their food sources and address problems with the immune system at the same time. The food sources for most of the organisms are heavy metals, iron, sugars, and foods that turn into sugar in the digestive process.

Yeast

There are different strains of candida, and it is normal to find it in the intestines and some in your mouth as well. It is a regular part of our bodies and is beneficial to a healthy body, aiding in digestion and nutrient absorption.

The healthy bacteria in your gut keep the candida levels in check. It's only when those good bacteria are disrupted or wiped out for some reason, or when there is too much food provided for candida, that fungal yeast infections develop. Then, candida can get out of hand.

Antibiotics can wipe out enough good bacteria to upset the balance in the digestive tract. Just one round of antibiotics can severely disrupt your microbiome and create a candida problem, which is why, many times, if you're given an antibiotic, you're also given an antifungal to take.

Other issues that can cause a problem with candida are high alcohol intake and a high-stress lifestyle.

There are some common symptoms of candida overgrowth:

- Skin rashes
- Nail fungal infections
- Feeling tired
- Digestive upset
- Autoimmune issues
- Brain fog
- Mood swings
- Allergies
- Sensitivity to smells

Any of the above could be a sign that you are having issues with candida.

There are steps to defeating candida. Attempting to eliminate this kind of overgrowth can be complicated. It can invade many parts of the body. We know that if we find that someone has an immune response to it in their blood upon IgG testing, it is indicative of a leaky gut because it doesn't belong in the bloodstream. We address candida not only with supplements that can help knock it back, but also with diet. There are certain dietary changes that need to be made to address candida.

One of the biggest problems with people who have candida is they are ingesting too much sugar, alcohol, or carbohydrates, like starchy grains and certain potatoes. These will all feed candida, so dietary changes will be necessary. Nuts may aggravate this condition for some people. We named gut-healing foods earlier.

Bacteria

There are several ways that a bacterial infection can present itself. Some types of bacteria can overgrow in the colon or in the small intestine (SIBO), which is when bacteria normally found in the lower large intestine or colon move into the upper small intestine where they don't belong. Candida overgrowth can be found along with either of these conditions.

Colon overgrowth is extremely common and can be identified by blood tests. It is important that we look carefully at your CBC (complete blood count). Medical professionals often ignore these tests when people show high lymphocyte, monocyte, or neutrophil counts or a chronic low white blood cell count. I often sit with people who have been told that those results are normal for them. When we dig deeper, we often find they have hidden bacterial overgrowth or dysbiosis (imbalanced gut flora).

Side note: infection can also be hidden in your dental work. If you have had a tooth extraction or a root canal, you should ask for a special X-ray, a 3D cone beam, to check for hidden infection in your jaw. Teeth are associated with meridians that connect them to the many organs and tissues of the body. Keeping a dead tooth (root canal) in your mouth has been correlated with disease in the organs on the same meridian as that tooth. This is regardless of if there is an infection visible on the 3D CT cone beam. A biological dentist would be best to help you determine your needs.

Some of those overgrown bacteria are bad bacteria, and we need to get them under control. Gut bacteria send signals— chemical messengers—to other parts of the body. Overgrowth of these bad bacteria, the more virulent strains of bacteria, are connected to conditions like Crohn's and ulcerative colitis. There are certain bacteria that can be associated with malignancies. This cannot be ignored. We can also associate bad bacteria with mental issues like being bipolar, having mood disorders, and autism.

We are learning a lot about our microbiome right now, and I do believe these kinds of studies will become even more important as we learn about the microbiome and its impact on our health and bodily functions.

Although bacteria belong in the colon, having an overgrowth of certain strains is a sign that the immune system is not able to keep things in check. It tells us some changes need to be made to knock that bacteria down and build up the good bacteria and the immune system. It tells us we need to shift the microbiome so the beneficial bacteria can outweigh the bad.

Parasites

You can get parasites walking barefoot. You can get parasites from your pets if they lick your face or sleep in bed with you. You can get them from eating raw meats, fish, or fruits and vegetables. We live in America, so we feel like we're not exposed; we think people need to go to a developing country to be exposed to parasites, but we are just as easily exposed here as anywhere. They are way more common than we realize.

Parasites may be harder to find on lab tests than other bugs. Sometimes there are indications, such as very high or very low iron counts, high eosinophils, monocytes, or basophils. Parasitic worms might be present; however, they don't always get found, even on a stool test. For some infections, you must catch a larva or an egg to find it. The smaller one-cell organisms that people get are easier to find. Newer DNA testing that may help us identify these issues is now available.

Parasites can express themselves with digestive issues such as persistent diarrhea, constipation, gas, skin issues, muscle aches, and joint pain. Many times, candida is also found when parasites are present. Parasites can cause inflammatory responses in the body.

We have different techniques we use to help eliminate parasites. The process is not always fun, but the health benefits that result when you heal your body from parasite infection are always well worth it. It is important to address not only the parasites but also any other associated health issues. We are often working on multiple layers when it comes to reducing inflammation from these bad bugs in the body.

One complicating factor is that heavy metals are food for parasites. Parasites and some bacteria tend to live on metals like iron. If the iron numbers are high or low, along with certain white blood cells, parasites or inflammation may be causing it. Iron levels can also be affected by heavy metal toxicity, so simply taking iron pills is merely a symptom treatment.

It's important to find out why the levels are too high or too low. The body could hoard iron to protect it. The body has an innate wisdom, and it knows what to do to protect itself at all costs. It will adapt.

As you can see, addressing these issues can be complicated. There may be multiple factors to look at. We need to build up the body, and at the same time, we need to try to kill off the overgrowing bugs.

For killing, we have a variety of herbal formulas, natural oils, and other remedies. We will often use nutraceuticals that are *synergistic*, meaning that they work together better than they work alone. Email me at drnicole@drnicole.com, and I will email you back a free parasite questionnaire.

There are different treatments for different problems. For candida, some of my favorites are oregano oil, garlic, and tea tree oil. For bacteria, there are several different formulas. There are formulas that contain black walnut and raspberry leaf and goldenseal, often combined with herbs, like Echinacea, that help build up the immune system. Garlic and oregano oil are beneficial. Beta-glucan is helpful in supporting the immune system. We work on bringing inflammation down with herbs like *curcumin.*

For parasites, formulas containing *mimosa pudica* are very effective. It is very sticky and helps drag them out. *Artemisinin* and wormseed oil are also useful. All of these remedies need to be used with caution. People will respond in a variety of ways. For some people, it's easy, and for some, it's more challenging. It's always best to work with someone who knows how to guide you through this process as gently as possible.

> *I have been a member of Rothman Health program now for some three months. It is a very comprehensive, carefully planned and developed program, covering all aspects of health and wellness. Dr. Nicole's approach is on finding the root cause for what is ailing you, analyzing thoroughly, and then planning a program to address the issues. The tests and analyses are thorough and treatment [is] tailored for you. Some two years ago, I started my own health journey to heal myself from an autoimmune disease that I had suffered with for over ten years. I achieved some positive results on my own following a special*

diet; however, that lifestyle—focusing only on diet— created other new health problems. After finding Dr. Nicole, I am now convinced that you need coaching and professional help and expertise in holistic wellness, and that is where Dr. Nicole and her staff are greatest. I can warmly recommend this program to anyone interested in improving their health and developing a sustainable, healthy lifestyle.

~ Riitta Rinttila

BUILDING UP THE BODY

As we previously mentioned, we shouldn't simply kill off whatever bad bugs might be overgrown in the gut and stop there.

We also need to work on:

- Building up the immune system
- Enhancing the body's ability to fight off different bugs
- Increasing the body's nutrient supply
- Promoting healing
- Replacing any deficiencies such as digestive enzymes

Repair Supplements

One of the best supplements is also one of my favorite foods: bone broth. Bone broth[5] has collagen and L-glutamine, which are two of the best supplements for helping to heal the gut. For reducing inflammation, we can use aqueous humic substances like *terrahydrite,* found in Ion Biome™. Curcumin, quercetin, marshmallow root, slippery elm, and aloe are all soothing for the gut. Apple cider vinegar is helpful for digestive purposes.

I also like using immunoglobulins to help repair the gut lining's first line of defense, secretory IgA (sIgA). It basically mimics the process of tightening the gut junctions while breastfeeding as an infant.

Proper digestion of fats, carbohydrates, and proteins requires adequate levels of different digestive enzymes. Many people who are dealing with gut issues are not making enough enzymes or hydrochloric acid to digest their food. In order to get properly digested food down into the small intestine and large intestine, we may have to work with the upper digestion in the stomach and use digestive enzymes to help those people.

In addition, supplementing with certain vitamins, like vitamins A, C, and D, as well as minerals like zinc, might

---

5 One of my healing *supplements* is actually a food and is my favorite: bone broth.

be necessary to boost the immune system. Vitamin D is best provided by safe sun exposure.

It's not just about building back the intestinal barrier, however. It's also necessary to build up the immune system by building up that good microbiome. When we eat, we want to consider our microbiome's needs too. Prebiotics, as we've discussed, are foods that feed your good bacteria. Chicory root and asparagus are two examples. Note that prebiotics are not the same as probiotics, which we will discuss in the next section.

Some other ways to support the intestinal mucosa are making sure we have enough short-chain fatty acids in the gut, and adding in l-glutamine, collagen, and aqueous humic substances like *Ion Biome*, which can help the tight junctions heal. These are all beneficial in getting that gut to tighten back up and become more adaptable again, to be a more welcoming environment to all our good microbiome species.

Rebalancing With Probiotics

One of the other ways we work to build up our health is by taking *probiotics*, which are beneficial microbes that will help shift your microbiome to a healthier state.

You might already know probiotics are helpful, but like most people, you may not know know how to choose the best ones for you. Most people have no idea what types of probiotics to take, how many are enough, how to determine quality, and how to determine if they are still viable by the time they get all the way down to your gut.

Probiotics are extremely important for us. Years ago, I attended a seminar and Dr. Steve Marini was the instructor. He said, "If you had the choice between a multivitamin and a probiotic, take the probiotic. Those good bacteria help you utilize and absorb vitamins and nutrients. They have their own antibiotic built into them. They are there to help us and support us. There are more of them than there are of us, so we should be feeding them."

There are different types of probiotics you can take as supplements. They may come in capsule form or liquid form. It's best to vary your probiotics and rotate through all the different types. Three of the most important ones are *bifidobacteria, lactobacillus,* and *Saccharomyces boulardii*[6] and *Bacillus* strains.

Bifidobacteria aid the immune system, help break nutrients down, and protect us from bad bacteria. Lactobacillus strains help us absorb nutrients, break down milk sugars, and produce lactic acid, which helps in muscle repair. Bacillus strains are soil organisms and are spore-forming, and these are highly resistant to our digestive enzymes. Lastly, the beneficial yeast *Saccharomyces boulardii* can help with fungal yeast infections.

---

6 There is a great deal of research on your gut microbiome right now so as time passes, we will probably learn that there are more microorganisms that are helpful in strengthening the microbiome.

These are specific strains we can send through our body. Just passing them through our digestive tract creates a wave of change in our own bacterial, fungal, and viral organisms that comprise our microbiome. This wave can shift our inner ecology into a healthier state.

When rotating through different strains, you want to be taking a minimum of 50 billion. You want to research to make sure they are viable and successfully getting into your body, but it is okay to cycle different levels or to even cycle on and off and just focus on fermented foods for some time. We want to try to find viable formulas that are very high in number because the higher the number, the more likely most of them travel down to where they belong.

You can rotate the dosage as well. You might pick one that is 50 billion one month, and another month, take one that is 100 billion, and then go back down to 50. Every now and then, I will take one that is 350 billion. You want to try to have an influx of different strains or even 20 or 30 and different viability. Try different companies as well. Listen to your body. Some might work better than others. But the one thing you don't want to do is stay on the same one for months or years at a time. That is not going to have any benefit in the long run.

In addition, we want to try the gut-healing foods I mentioned earlier in this book: the sauerkrauts, kimchi, kefir waters, kefir-cultured, raw dairy products, and kombucha. Consider feeding your microbiome on a daily basis, and you will enhance the good flora of your body.

Eliminating the cause of the damage is an obvious strategy. Getting off medications, learning better lifestyle strategies, reducing stress, cutting out unnatural and destructive foods, getting more exercise, and sleeping well will all help.

The Microbiome

The microbiome that exists in our bodies has been the subject of many research studies in recent years. You're going to hear more and more about the microbiome as the research results come out.

What exactly is this microbiome?

It consists of a gigantic community of microorganisms: bacteria, fungi, viruses, and even parasites, if you have them. They live in and on our bodies, and we can't function properly without them.

We begin to develop our microbiome even before we're born. The stress your mother experienced while you were in her womb could affect your microbiome because you may have stress hormones and stress responses that affect it. The way that you're born affects your microbiome; if you're born by C-section, you're going to have a different microbiome than if you're born vaginally. The exposure the baby experiences to the mother's bacteria in the passage through the birth canal is what we call *the first meal*. That first exposure starts the process of building the baby's new, healthy microbiome.

Breastfeeding will affect how a baby's microbiome develops and how their gastrointestinal barrier develops, as will medications during the first years of life, like vaccinations and antibiotics. We are born with a leaky gut. Immunoglobulins found in colostrum and breastfeeding close up the tight junctions and allow a healthy gut barrier. If a baby is being fed solid foods before their body is ready, this could be a potential cause of health issues, such as digestive distress, inflammation, or food allergies.

If you've had emotional difficulties in your childhood, or specific traumas, these can impact your microbiome; stress has a major impact on it. If you're eating a lot of GMO foods, soda, or other unhealthy foods as you're growing up, these are all things that can impact you as you're developing and maturing.

When we look at children, we often aren't as concerned about their diets as we should be.

We think: *Oh, you're just a kid. You don't need to eat healthy. Kids can get away with anything.*

However, diet is important. It impacts us as we're developing, as we're maturing.

There are 360 times more genes in your microbiome. That means when you count up all the genes of the bacteria, fungi, viruses, and all kinds of organisms in your microbiome, there are 360 times more genes in your microbiome than in your body. The way we treat our bodies, we have to wonder who is really living on whom. Maybe we are there to feed them rather than they are here to feed us. We're learning that they are way more important than we ever realized.

We must pay attention to our microbiome and nourish it. To maintain our own health, we need to feed our microbiome and take care of it. We know that it has a huge impact on the development of disease. There are connections between our microbiome and obesity, heart disease, diabetes, mood and emotional states, hormone health, and our immune system. This microbiome plays roles in many parts of our health and our lives.

As research comes out, we are going to find it is even more important than we imagined. Microorganisms are here on this earth, and they are not going anywhere. Attacking these organisms is not the path to health. We need them. They are an integral part of being human and being on this planet. Until we understand they are life forms necessary for us to be alive, we can never understand what real health is.

We also need to look at our lifestyles carefully to assess what is damaging our bodies. When it comes to rebuilding the gut, we can't forget about the factors that damaged it in the first place.

Here are some questions to ask yourself:

- *Am I too sedentary?*
- *Am I under a great deal of physical stress?*
- *Am I suffering from lack of sleep?*
- *Am I on a lot of medications?*
- *What chemicals am I exposed to on a daily basis?*
- *Am I cleaning my house with Clorox wipes all the time?*
- *What level of emotional stress am I under?*
- *Am I consuming too much alcohol?*
- *How much TV do I watch?*
- *How exposed am I to EMFs?*

We should look at all the different sources of body tissue damage to see what is tearing us down while we are trying to build ourselves up.

This can be done. It doesn't happen overnight. When you wipe out the bad, build up the good, and heal the tissues that have been damaged, you can absolutely heal your body, heal your gut, and turn chronic degenerative disease and acute problems around.

CHAPTER FOUR

Nutrition for Life

WHAT IS FOOD?

What is food anyway?

The actual definition of food, according to the Macmillan dictionary, is: "That which is eaten to sustain life, provide energy, and promote growth and repair of the tissues."

Most of us think food is just something to fill our bellies, to satisfy our emotional cravings, or to relieve boredom. We may see food as primarily related to social engagements and activities. In actuality, food is a building block for our body. Its purpose is to give us the energy and the materials to build and create new tissue, to provide nutrients that we require, and ultimately, to sustain our lives.

Fats, Proteins, and Carbohydrates

Instead of worrying about how much to eat all day long and how many calories to consume, we need to learn the right food to eat and the right time to eat it. Most people focus on calorie counting as a way to get healthy, but that won't help you heal your body, lose weight, or optimize your well-being. You need to develop an understanding of the different types of food in order to determine what foods are best for your body, to heal it and to help it function at your highest potential level.

There are three different types of macronutrients in foods. They are fats, proteins, and carbohydrates.

Fat is a good source of energy as opposed to some of the other foods we eat. Fat provides nine calories per gram. However, some types of fats may not be very good for us because they are inflammatory. Healthy fats can be found in foods like avocados, coconut oil, olive oil, nuts, and seeds. These foods are high in fats, especially the raw, organic ones. We can also get healthy fats from grass-fed meats and wild-caught cold-water fish.

Protein comes from meat, fish, and poultry, but there are vegetable proteins as well, in foods like beans and soy. It's also important that we understand that protein is not as good a source of energy as fat; it only provides four calories per gram.

Carbohydrates are what most people think of when they think of getting energy. It is what we often look for when we are grabbing a snack, usually a sugary or starchy something to give us energy. Carbohydrates include grains, sweet potatoes, white potatoes and sugars, as well as refined carbohydrates like pasta and bread. Carbohydrates, like proteins, only give us four calories per gram. Vegetables and fruits are also carbohydrates, but the body processes them differently than the starchy carbs like corn and potatoes—they cause the highest spikes of insulin.

The calorie is a unit of energy. Fat has the most units of energy per gram—nine. We want our body to be using fat for energy instead of carbohydrates, which break down into glucose in the body. Most people with metabolic or health issues, energy, sleep, or blood sugar issues are burning glucose instead of fat for energy. You want to get the body to convert into a fat burner instead of a sugar burner. This is how you will heal your metabolic issues.

How do you get the body to convert from a sugar burner to a fat burner?

You train it to look for fat. If you never ran a marathon, you would train before running one. If you are always consuming things that are quick sources of glucose—the carbohydrates—then your body is going to look for and crave those foods. We must take them away so that the body looks for fats instead. We do that by eliminating starchy carbohydrates and fruit and increasing fat intake so the body doesn't have much of a choice.

During this process, you will be creating a metabolic shift in your body that will become a significant advantage for you. Sometimes changing your diet in this way requires a transitional period during which you may not feel as well. This happens when there is little glucose for the brain to utilize and it isn't using ketones released from fat to function yet. However, if you are giving the body the proper amounts of nutrients during this process, it usually doesn't take that long to adjust. It's generally very easy to make this metabolic shift.

Mother Nature: The Way Food Was Before Humans Got Their Hands on It

When we think about the foods found in nature, we usually think about foods that are grown in the ground, foods that come out of the soil. That is what most people think of vegetables and fruit. However, there are foods found in nature that we have altered, such as some meats, dairy, and vegetables.

We need to understand the same power that created Planet Earth and all the wonderful resources on it is the same power that created us. We must recognize that the more we toil with what has been created for us naturally, and the more altered it becomes, the harder it is for our body to process it. Seek out the foods that are naturally needed by us. When you get back to those roots, your body can start to heal.

You may have heard this saying:

> *If your great-grandmother didn't eat it,*
> *you probably shouldn't be eating it either.*

It is true. We need to get back to how earlier generations used to eat. They ate loads of real food. They ate clean fruits and vegetables that were not altered with genetic modifications, foods that were not mass-produced and processed. People grew their own food more often. They had their own gardens and farms. They relied on the land to provide their nutrients for them. Food can heal and help us Awaken Wellness.

Since the sixties, our soil has been depleted of a lot of the nutrients we need. That is why so many of us need to take supplements. It would be wiser—and much more affordable—if we could get these nutrients from our food sources. That was how it was designed in the first place.

We need to get back to the basics and understand that the more we stop looking to advances in agriculture, the more we get back to natural ways like growing our own food or finding farmers who use natural practices to farm the food for us, the better our health is going to be. It will make a huge difference.

How Often Do We Really Need to Eat?

Eliminating toxins from your food and your lifestyle will probably be one of the most important pieces in regaining your health. When you reduce the toxic load in your body, you will improve your ability to absorb nutrients, which will increase your body's ability to restore and regenerate healthy, new tissue.

People think that *grazing*—eating several small meals a day—is the best way to be healthy. I have worked with many diabetics who had been told to eat all day to keep their blood sugar up, but this is exactly the opposite of what they need to do to heal. It is exactly why so many are remaining diabetic no matter how much weight they lose or how hard they try.

I have been in the fitness environment since I was seventeen years old, and I had always been told to eat five to seven meals a day. We were told to have snacks in between to keep our blood sugar levels normalized. However, we now know that these eat-all-day diets are a huge mistake.

Why is this grazing strategy a mistake?

Every time we eat, no matter what we eat, our body must process the food. As a result, insulin is going to spike. Part of the metabolic challenges our generation is facing today is from eating not only the wrong foods, but eating them way too often. It is not a proportion or a calorie issue for the most part. The timing of how we eat is going to be one of the most important tools in shifting this metabolism.

Insulin spikes can contribute to the development of *insulin resistance*—when the body cells cease to respond to insulin the way they were designed to. We should allow longer periods of insulin to be maintained at low levels in order to desensitize the cells and stop resistance.

The strategy of creating long periods without food is called *intermittent fasting*. Fasting goes back to ancient times. It's still part of many religious practices. For instance, I fast every single year on Yom Kippur. It used to be one of the most miserable days of the entire year, but now it's no big deal because I've trained my body to go without food for longer periods of time. When your body is trained to use fat for energy, you can go a long time without food, even if you're exercising, working, and being active. When you notice this, you will know your body has a better metabolism.

The first step in making this shift is trying to stretch that fasting period out naturally. Start by fasting after dinner until breakfast. Breakfast, after all, actually means *break the fast*.

Next, try eating just three meals a day: breakfast, lunch, and dinner, with no snacks whatsoever. If you can do this, it is a huge accomplishment. It can be difficult because you may get cravings at night, or you may get very hungry in the middle of the day. You need to train your body to stretch that window in which you are not spiking insulin.

The next step, when you feel comfortable with this, is to try to skip breakfast and not eat until lunch, allowing for a longer period without insulin spiking. We have been told that breakfast is the most important meal of the day, and for some people, it might be. It could be better for you to skip dinner instead. Pushing the body is how you are going to train and strengthen so many body functions, whether it is through exercising, or by how often and at what time of day you're eating.

You can begin gradually. Drop your usual early breakfast and see how long you can go before eating. Take a week or two to see if you can push it, go to ten o'clock in the morning, then eleven o'clock, then noon. You will shift your metabolism much faster and heal the parts of you that need help.

Eventually, when you are skipping that first meal, you can jump ahead to skipping maybe the whole day of eating. You might want to try not eating until dinner one day a week. That is a twenty-four-hour fast. Eventually you can build up to an extended fast. That would be ideal for many.

You don't want to create a fixed routine. Diet variation is key. We don't want to let the body become too familiar with what we're doing. Maybe you skip breakfast five days a week. Maybe you fast a full day and skip breakfast and lunch, so you don't eat until dinnertime one day a week. Then maybe that other day, that seventh day, you eat from the moment you wake up. You eat three meals and start in the morning. You can lower your fat intake and increase your carb or protein intake these days. That is called diet variation.

When you become experienced with intermittent fasting, you can start to stretch and flex your metabolic muscle. Some will jump right into a five-day fast. Perhaps you will see if you can go for thirty-six hours, then forty-eight, until you build up to the ideal five days or more. You can fast without food and only water, you can do a bone broth fast, or you can do a fasting-mimicking diet, such as Prolon™, that packages the exact foods for you to eat in a five-day window. I advise that if you do one of these longer-term fasts, you have someone who knows what they're doing supervising you, helping you structure your food correctly in order to safely manage this type of advanced fasting. Fasting helps you see the power of your innate intelligence.

WHAT ISN'T FOOD?

There are a lot of *food-like* items out there that people think are foods, but are they?

Consider the little chunks of processed meat with glue in between them, and the highly processed snacks and meals that are composed primarily of fillers, additives, and artificial fats.

Are these truly foods?

No, they are not, according to our definition of food. They do not provide nutrients. They may provide energy, but they are definitely not going to help us grow and repair our tissues.

These heavily processed foods are some of the cheapest foods available to us. Unfortunately, they're often more affordable than healthy foods. We've created a culture of fast-food eaters out of necessity. Our kids are eating fast foods several times a week partly because they have a dollar menu available to them.

These food-like items are destructive to our tissues. They deliver the exact opposite of growing and repairing our tissues. We have sicker children than we have ever seen in our history. It is estimated that one out of three children who were born after the year 2000 will develop diabetes.[7] We must show our children what food really is. We must understand that if we as adults don't make different choices, we'll be watching the demise of the human race from this one crisis alone.

We need to talk with each other and our children about what is not food. We need to talk about what we don't want to put in our bodies, as well as what we want to put in them. Making these choices is taking our power back to control our health and Awaken Wellness.

Frankenfood

Many of us remember Frankenstein movies: the story about how a mad scientist created a so-called person in a lab. The person ended up being a monster. That is how I look at these human-made foods, these *frankenfoods* that are lab-created, that are not made by Mother Nature. These

7 Narayan, K.M. Venkat, et. al. "Lifetime Risk for Diabetes Mellitus in the United States." *Jama Network.* 08 October 2003. Doi:10.1001/jama.290.14.1884

foods are genetically altered for many different reasons: to prevent bugs from eating them, to increase yield, to improve appearance, and to lengthen shelf life.

We know there are studies proving these frankenfoods are causing cancer and obesity, all kinds of mental-diminishing diseases, Parkinson's, Alzheimer's,[8] problems with fertility,[9] allergies, depression, cardiovascular diseases,[10] and neurodegenerative diseases.

Pesticides are also impacting food quality. Glyphosate, a chemical that is commonly used—in products like *Round Up*—to kill weeds and prevent bugs, is one of the biggest challenges we are dealing with. We are now seeing lawsuits filed by people who have developed lymphoma and other cancers after using glyphosate on a regular basis. It is likely we will be seeing more and more of these reports in the near future.

Frankenfoods are not foods you should put into your body. However, it is sometimes hard to determine which foods are natural foods in our markets. The food industry does not

---

8 Woodruff, Emily. "Processed Food Leads to Alzheimer's, Says Expert." *being patient.* 26 March 2018. beingpatient.com/processed-food-alzheimers/

9 Pultarova, Tereza. "How Eating Fast Food May Make It Harder to Get Pregnant." *LIVESCIENCE.* 03May 2018. livescience.com/62476-fast-food-diet-infertility.html

10 Srour, Bernard, et. al. "Ultra-processed food intake and risk of cardiovascular disease: prospective cohort study." *thebmj.* bmj.com/content/365/bmj.l11451

want to label foods with a GMO sticker; they do not want to tell people these are the foods that will make you sick.

There continue to be debates about requiring the labeling of GMO foods. Meanwhile, there have been other initiatives such as the Non-GMO Project. The Non-GMO project, dedicated to consumer education and outreach, is providing some labeling to those companies that are not using GMOs in products. Through this labeling system, we can see what foods are not GMO in our markets, so we can pick them instead.

Take the time to look for these Non-GMO labels. This is something we need to do to protect our bodies from contamination. We need to stop eating frankenfoods that can create chronic degenerative diseases. They are damaging to our long-term health.

Processed Foods and Artificial Ingredients

I'm not saying you can never eat processed foods again. Yes, we all live in a fast-paced lifestyle. I do as well. These foods are convenient and sometimes will come in handy, but we need to make good choices.

If you are using prepared foods, you want to make sure they are either organic or non-GMO. If something says it is organic, it cannot be a GMO food. However, non-GMO foods are not necessarily organic. We want to make sure that, minimally, we are choosing non-GMO food.

In addition, there are many food additives and chemicals that you want to avoid. Additives are used in food products as preservatives, fillers, or to artificially enhance texture, color, or flavor. There are many food additives that change the way food tastes to us. As a result, many people grow to think that healthy foods don't taste good, but junk food does. Initially, many people I work with will tell me that natural foods don't taste good to them. It's fascinating to me how their palates change as we work together to improve their health. As we work on detoxing, bettering their lifestyle and diet, natural foods begin to taste good. It's pretty amazing that when we start eliminating these chemicals from our diet and improving our microbiome, our taste preferences change too.

Read the lists of ingredients on your food but be aware that the same chemical might go by a few different names. To be safe, if there is an ingredient in a food that you don't recognize as a food substance, you might want to avoid that product.

Did you know they sometimes rename familiar chemicals on the labels?

For example, you may not see the ingredient *MSG (monosodium glutamate)* on a label, but be aware that *autolyzed yeast, L-glutamic acid,* and *hydrolyzed vegetable proteins* are names that actually mean MSG.

Some common additives we should avoid or minimize are:

- MSG
- Nitrites
- Hydrogenated and artificial fats
- Artificial sweeteners
- High fructose corn syrup
- Food coloring
- Food preservatives

MSG

MSG is an additive that alters the ability of your brain to know when you're full. You know the stories about eating Chinese food. When we eat Chinese food, we are often hungry an hour later. That is because they are notoriously famous for adding MSG to their sauces as a flavor enhancer, but as a result, your body has no idea that it's full. Those receptors are being shut off. MSG can also be addictive.

Nitrites

The World Health Organization told us years ago that processed meat with nitrites causes cancer, yet we are still making and eating them.[11]

---

11 World Health Organization. "IAR Monographs evaluate consumption of red meat and processed meat." 26 October 2015. iarc. fr/wp-content/uploads/2018/07/pr240_E.pdf

Hydrogenated and Artificial Fats

So many of us went along with the fat-free fad that started in the late 80's, which resulted in effectively destroying millions of people's metabolisms. Because everybody was going crazy eating carbs and being afraid of fats, the food industry began hydrogenating fats to make foods creamier so they would only have to add a little tiny bit of fat into a food product, and then they could say it was fat-free or low-fat. The liver has a hard time dealing with these hydrogenated fats, so they cannot be processed properly by the liver. These fats literally destroy your arteries.

Canola oil is in almost all processed foods. Just read the labels, even in the natural food stores. Canola is highly inflammatory and was originally used as a machine lubricant oil. It contains euric acid, a known carcinogen. However, trace amounts are allowed by the FDA. Reducing inflammation is an important aspect of staying well, so avoiding canola and other inflammatory oils is of huge benefit to your overall health and longevity.

Artificial Sweeteners

Artificial sweeteners should never have ever been allowed in our food supply. Aspartame accounts for over 75 percent of adverse reactions of all the food additives that are recorded in the FDA. Aspartame can cross the blood-brain barrier and can cause symptoms of fibromyalgia, Alzheimer's, chronic fatigue syndrome, multiple sclerosis (MS), memory loss, headaches, and weight gain.[12]

It is incredible how the food industry has changed the labeling so you don't know what's in there anymore. Then they promote artificial sweeteners like sucralose, also known as Splenda, which may be destructive to your good gut bacteria because it's chlorinated sugar. Chlorine is toxic to us.

High Fructose Corn Syrup

High fructose corn syrup is added to many processed foods. It is highly inflammatory. Keep in mind that, in general, sugar is inflammatory, even though it is a natural substance— Mercury has been found in small amounts of high fructose corn syrup. For a great documentary on the effects of sugar, I recommend watching *That Sugar Film*, directed by Damon Gameau (2015) and available on multiple platforms, including YouTube, Amazon Prime, and Google Play.

Food Coloring and Food Preservatives

Food colorings and preservatives such as BHT (butylated hydroxytoluene), TBHQ (tert-Butylhydroquinone), and others can have detrimental effects on your body.

---

12 Lillis, Charlotte. "What are the side effects of aspartame?" *Medical News Today*. 14 January 2019. medicalnewstoday.com/articles/322266. php

Many of these toxic additives are capable of damaging your cells. Your liver cannot process them, and they provide little nutritive value. If we want to use foods to heal our bodies, we need to avoid these additives. Remember, if there is a word you don't recognize on a label, or if it sounds off, you probably want to avoid it—even when it sounds healthy, like *hydrolyzed vegetable protein*. If you don't know what it is, you should not be eating it. Don't put your money there.

Spend your money on foods made by companies that make foods with a purpose. They care about people's health. They are willing to put on a non-GMO label and pay to be part of that project. They are willing to use farming practices to create foods that are better for you. They care about the environment. The extra fifty cents you're paying speaks volumes about the type of foods we are demanding in our country.

Human-made Meats, Dairy, and Vegetables

Suppose you are trying to eat healthy foods. You go to the grocery store and pick up some healthy vegetables in the produce section. You go over to the meat department and get some chicken or some ground low-fat meat. Then, you head over to the dairy department and get some yogurt to snack on because you've been told this is healthy. You select *Yoplait* or *Dannon* or one of the popular brands advertised on TV.

You bring your food purchases home, thinking you've avoided processed foods and stocked your cupboard with much healthier food choices.

How did you do? Are these foods the healthy choices you thought they were?

The yogurt probably is not. It is likely full of sugar and additives. Just read the labels. You will find flavors and artificial sweeteners galore. You might see too much sugar added. Also, conventional dairy is laden with hormones and antibiotics.

What about the meats?

We often can't be sure about the quality of meats, and this is a problem. We need absolute transparency when it comes to our food products.

Here are some questions we'd like answered:

- What were those animals given to eat?
- Were they given food that they would naturally have been eating if they were just out in the environment and not on a farm?
- In what environment were the animals raised?
- How was the meat processed?
- What chemicals, hormones, and antibiotics were the animals exposed to?

Conventional meat cattle are usually fed GMO grains, corn, and soy. However, if cattle were given the opportunity to eat a pile of grains or feed on a grassy field, they would naturally go to the grassy field. Their bodies are designed to digest those foods. Their digestive systems are different from ours. Our body isn't designed to digest those types of foods, but a cow's body is. When we give a person the wrong kinds of food, the person gets sick. When we give a cow the wrong type of food, the cow gets sick too.

Conventional meats are likely to have been mass-produced. The cows are shoved into a tightly packed area. They are stressed out and often have high cortisol as a result. They are in an environment where it's easy for them to get sick, so they are given massive amounts of antibiotics to prevent disease. They are given hormones to quickly grow the meat so producers can get it out to sell as fast as possible.

This is not natural food. These are human-made meats, not real foods. The meat is full of stress hormones, antibiotics, and growth hormones.

It's because of this industry that we currently have more problems with superbugs—the problem is due to all the antibiotics being put in these foods. Girls are developing and maturing earlier from the hormones in food. This is not okay. Of all antibiotics sold in the United States, approximately 80% are sold for use in animal agriculture.[13] They are not

---

13 Summary Report on Antimicrobials Sold or Distributed for Use

healthy. They are inflammatory. They won't be a good choice. They are going to make you sick.

We need to eat grass-fed, natural meats that haven't been injected with all kinds of chemicals. We should choose meat and dairy from animals that are allowed to roam freely and are not stressed out, and are eating healthy food, not food covered in chemicals or are genetically modified.

Typically, dairy products are heated, breaking them down and destroying any of its nutritive properties. Raw dairy has the most benefit because it contains all kinds of natural enzymes. However, you should be aware that even in its most natural form dairy could be inflammatory. Conventional dairy is from A1 genetic cows. Many people find that A2 cows are less inflammatory and allergenic, and they can tolerate these dairy products and enjoy their many benefits. However, many people can't tolerate dairy in any form.

When it comes to our vegetables, we have already talked about GMOs. You may not know if the vegetables you purchased are GMO because they are not necessarily labeled this way. You may be able to find an option labeled non-GMO in your produce section if you're lucky. Vegetables may also have chemical residue on them that can be unhealthy. A lot of our foods are being sprayed with all kinds of pesticides and

in Food-Producing Animals. 2014. Available at: http://www.fda.gov/downloads/ForIndustry/UserFees/AnimalDrugUsedFeeActADUFA/UCM338170.pdf. Accessed June 15, 2015.

chemicals to preserve them, and they are not being grown in healthy soil, so they don't contain the nutrients we need out of them.

> *Genetically modified organisms (GMOs) are living organisms whose genetic material has been artificially manipulated in a laboratory through genetic engineering. This creates combinations of plant, animal, bacteria, and virus genes that do not occur in nature or through traditional crossbreeding methods.*

> *Most GMOs have been engineered to withstand the direct application of herbicide or to produce an insecticide. However, new technologies are now being used to artificially develop other traits in plants, such as a resistance to browning in apples, and to create new organisms using synthetic biology. Despite biotech industry promises, there is no evidence that any of the GMOs currently on the market offer increased yield, drought tolerance, enhanced nutrition, or any other consumer benefit.[14]*

Just because it *looks* natural, doesn't mean it *is* natural. We need to ask more questions. We need to know how these foods have been grown. This is called transparency.

Selecting foods that are labeled *organic* is the best way to avoid GMOs and to use food to Awaken Wellness.

---

14 "GMO Facts." *Non-GMO Project.* https://www.nongmoproject.org/gmo-facts/

In the grocery store, I heard a little boy saying to his mom, as he picked up an organic cauliflower, "Mom, I heard picking organic is better."

She said, "Oh, that's just a lie. It's not true. It's just a lie to make more money."

I wanted to stop them and say, "That's what you're teaching the future generation? Is it okay to eat these bad foods that you have in your cart but not invest an extra dollar in a healthier vegetable?" We need to show our children they have the power to be healthy.

Yes, it is possible some food companies out there are lying in their marketing statements. However, you have a much better chance of getting something more natural and less contaminated when you buy organic than when you buy the conventional products we know are loaded with chemicals and medications.

We must make the effort to choose foods that are healing foods. When you eat grass-fed meats and pastured poultry, you're eating foods that can help you heal. They won't be inflammatory. They won't make you have heart attacks and heart disease. They are the natural foods we are meant to eat.

NEVER AGAIN

After you drop some foods from your diet to begin the process of becoming healthier, you will have to make some decisions about the path you're going to take to Awaken Wellness.

Sometimes, when I am teaching people about what to eat, I will say, "You should never add this back into your diet again," and they look at me in horror and shock.

They don't really understand why this is so important. When you make a decision that your health is your number one priority, and you are trying to make your life the best life possible, there are just certain things you're going to need to eliminate. We want to get well and STAY WELL.

The first one I advocate is: *Never again add refined sugars into your diet.*

Does this mean you can never have a birthday cake again?

Of course, you can have a birthday cake on your birthday, but you can pick a healthier version of what you enjoy. We can make smart choices so that even that one day a year—it's okay to splurge every now and then—we can make a choice that is not going to destroy us for three, four, five days afterward.

Once you get your body clean, you will see how poorly it reacts to these foods. It will be obvious. We can advise you *never again,* but you might need to learn the hard way, by experimenting. Once you eliminate a food and eat it again, you will see how negatively it affects you; sometimes, you may feel the effects for a whole week afterward.

Soon, you will find yourself saying: *I am never eating that again.* It's just not worth it.

Our basic *never again* list includes:

- Refined sugars
- Artificial sugar substitutes
- Gluten
- Soy
- Bad oils—we will explain below

Some of you will add dairy and grains to this list.

Sugar and Artificial Sweeteners

One of the most damaging substances you can ingest is sugar, in particular, the refined sugars we see in most foods. The average American consumes about thirty-two teaspoons of sugar every single day. Sugar is extremely inflammatory. It creates insulin resistance, weight gain, and liver damage.

Sugar feeds the bad bugs we talked about earlier. It can fuel yeast overgrowth, bacterial overgrowth, and dysbiosis, where bacterial balance in the body is thrown off. It can cause metabolic dysfunction, where the body is constantly looking for sugar for energy. You can have some serious ups and downs throughout the day when you are dependent on sugar for body processes.

Sugar feeds cancer cells. It promotes cell division and cancer growth, allowing it to spread faster. It's highly addictive, acting on the same part of the brain as cocaine.

There are studies that show that sugar actually makes you dumb.[15] It makes you dumber. There is a UCLA study where rats were first given a regular diet. They were put through a maze that they had to figure out. Then they added high fructose corn syrup into their diet. They found it slowly hampered the brain, memory, and learning. They saw that the rats could no longer figure out how to get through the maze. They were bumping into each other. They were acting differently. Their behavior totally changed. It was completely disrupted.

It's obvious that it's a problem for humans too. We have more learning disabilities, behavioral issues, and mood issues than we have ever seen in history, and we have more sugar in our diet than ever before.

When my practice members give up sugar, some have withdrawal symptoms. People feel horrible sometimes, but after a couple of days, they begin to feel better. Those energy ups and downs they used to have go away. They have better moods, less anxiety, and less depression. It's totally worth it!

We have already discussed artificial sweeteners. Replacing sugar with artificial sweeteners is a bad idea. Most people do this to lose their weight, or if they are diabetic, they may be told not to eat sugar, so they replace it with an artificial

---

15 "This is your brain on sugar: UCLA study shows high-fructose diet sabotages learning, memory." *UCLA Health.* 15 May 2012. uclahealth. org/high-fructose-diet-sabotages-learning-memory

sweetener. These artificial sugar replacements are chemicals that alter the way your body functions, and not in a good way.

My favorite natural replacement for sugar, and to help with sugar cravings, is extract from the stevia plant. You can also use non-GMO monk fruit, but I like stevia extract the most. You always want to try to stick with organic stevia. Try to avoid the most popular stevias such as Truvia, which Pepsi makes, because it contains GMO corn powder. You really need to know what you're selecting.

I like liquid stevia extracts because they are not made with any powders, and they have the least opportunity to be altered. Whenever we extract from an herb, it's usually going to be in liquid form, so this form will be the purest and least processed.

Stevia can be helpful for you as you are eliminating sugar because you may experience cravings. It really does taste good if you can find the right one. It won't taste exactly like sugar, but your taste buds will adapt.

Gluten and Soy

Everybody knows about gluten now, but just a few years ago, nobody even knew what it was. Back in 1999, I read a book called *Eat Right 4 Your Blood Type*, by Peter D'Adamo, and it said that, for my blood type, wheat and gluten were not good. I stopped eating gluten then, and it made a drastic difference. It was amazing what it did for me in just a couple of weeks. I'd had some acne during my pregnancy and for many years. My skin cleared up in two weeks after years of acne, and I learned the value of eliminating gluten.

The grains of today are not like the ancient grains; our bodies don't process them as well as they used to. You can learn how we started eating these grasses to begin with and how inflammatory they were for us through some wonderful resources out there. Many of my practice members see that grains are some of the most inflammatory foods for them, gluten in particular. Many people cannot tolerate gluten anymore and many feel better when they avoid it. The addition of glyphosate to the harvesting process is fueling the fire and our bodies can't tolerate the chemical burden.

Soy is another problem food. These two foods are so prevalent in the Standard American Diet—abbreviated SAD, interestingly enough. Soy is estrogenic. That means it can act like an estrogen in the body. For our males, this is not ideal. For females, estrogen dominance is highly correlated with different female cancers.

Soy, corn, and wheat gluten, unless organic, are going to be GMO foods. They are going to be frankenfoods and extremely inflammatory. We know that gluten is one of the most damaging foods to our gut lining. Leaky gut is a huge problem for people. If we can avoid soy and gluten, we should. Luckily, these days, it is very easy to find replacements for gluten. There are a lot of gluten-free processed foods out there. We have two bakeries in our town, both gluten free, and one is vegan as well. They are using non-GMO foods. They are transparent when it comes to all their ingredients. Great for treats!

Be aware that a lot of gluten-free foods are not health foods. They are just using the labeling for marketing. Read the ingredients. They may add corn and other fillers like tapioca to make the product stick together. Gluten is like a glue. It helps things stick together. They need to find something else to do that.

Many gluten-free products also have sugar added, and you may find soy oil or soy lecithin. These are highly inflammatory, often rancid, and commonly found in processed foods.

Avoiding gluten and soy can be tricky when eating out, and you can create your own problem-solving strategies. We will go out for sushi every once in a blue moon. I am not promoting sushi because there are issues with fish and heavy metals and radiation. However, on the rare occasions that we go, we bring our own coconut aminos because the soy sauce in these restaurants will absolutely have GMO gluten and GMO soy in it.

You will create your own strategies for eating out, deciding where your limits are and what you are going to allow for yourself.

If you do eat gluten, pay attention to how you're feeling. If you have eliminated it for a while, carefully note how you feel. Your body will tell you what's right for you and what isn't.

Bad Oils

Bad oils are oils that are extremely inflammatory. The body cannot process them. Many of the oils you're being exposed to when you go out to eat or are in processed foods are rancid. Oils are very delicate; the process of making the oil to put in a bottle can create a rancid, inflammatory substance. Most of the restaurants that fry foods are using the same oils repeatedly. This includes donuts, french fries, and other fried foods. These are all oils that can damage your heart, arteries, liver. They bog down your entire system and are extremely inflammatory.

Fats are important. We need them to heal, as we spoke about earlier.

How do we solve the problem of adding healthy fats into our diet?

We want to make sure the oils we're using are the right types of oil, and that they're not rancid. We want to make sure they are cold-pressed instead of heated so we are not consuming an already-damaged oil. It's also better in a dark bottle so light is not oxidizing it.

You will also want to stay away from oils such as canola, corn, soybean, vegetable, and sunflower oils, which are in everything these days. These are an absolute *do not buy*. They're in almost all the processed foods.

One of the biggest problems with highly processed, industrial oils, like corn, soybean, sunflower, and canola is that the polyunsaturated component of the oil is highly unstable under heat, light, and pressure. These elements heavily oxidize the polyunsaturates, creating free radicals in your body. The end result of all this refining and processing are oils that are highly inflammatory in your body when you ingest them, causing potential weight gain, heart disease, strokes, and other degenerative disease.

We also want to avoid hydrogenated oils, the completely human-made oils that are in 42 percent of regular foods in the grocery store. They're in 95 percent of cookies, 75 percent of chips and crackers, cold cereals, frozen breakfast foods, and almost all microwave popcorn.

You should say no to these bad oils. Choose restaurants that use oils you approve. This is not easy to find. Sometimes, I bring my own coconut oil with me when I go out, because it's not so easy to find, so I can have items steamed and add my own oil. I don't eat the salad dressing because I don't know what kind of oil is in it. I'll ask for olive oil. At least it's better than vegetable oil, which is probably what's in the salad dressing.

We need to use these problem-solving strategies when we're traveling and eating away from home. Bring your own foods when necessary. When I travel, I bring coconut oil and MCT (medium-chain triglyceride) oil with me so I know I have a healthy oil in my hotel room. I will throw an avocado in my bag. Bring one with you so you're prepared.

You must say *no* and *never again* to these foods: the sugars, the artificial sweeteners, gluten, soy, and these bad oils. If you simply cut these particular foods out of your diet, you can drastically change your state of health for the better.

> *What I especially love about Dr. Nicole Rothman is she absolutely cares with her heart and soul about the success of her people . . . she will do anything to ensure you are making progress and succeeding in your goals. Not only that, Dr. Nicole Walks the Talk! She truly believes in healthy and organic in every aspect of her and your lifestyle. There is nobody that is more dedicated than Dr. Nicole. She is a True Inspiration to me and I am very grateful to her! Troy, the office manager, and Natalie, my great coach, are pure delights to work with and are smiling and happy all the time. Thank you for everything you all do! I highly recommend Dr. Nicole and her fantastic staff!*
> ~ Paula Fredette

CHAPTER FIVE

The Power

MOVEMENT

We need to find ways to connect body, mind, and soul. We tend to disconnect from our body. We have been told our body is bad and to ignore how it feels. When our body has symptoms, we are told to shut them down, to suppress them with medications. We have not learned to trust our body or to have faith in a natural healing process, which can be uncomfortable at times.

It is important to develop a connection to your body again and recognize your body is a messenger. A lot of your brain energy goes into processing movement and allowing you to maintain your body's relationship with gravity. You want to make sure you are using movement in a positive way.

In order for you to embrace your power, you need to become self-aware, and movement is a key factor in creating self-awareness. Regular body movement has a multitude of beneficial effects on the body.

We have listed some of them below:

- Activates the brain
- Promotes self-awareness and other-awareness
- Fosters interaction between people
- Reduces stress
- Protects us from injury
- Develops flexibility
- Releases happy hormones and endorphins
- Creates better spatial awareness
- Improves athletic ability
- Boosts our mental health
- Helps us feel good

Fitness

When it comes to exercise, we need to recognize there are a lot of different ways we can achieve a level of fitness. One thing I always caution people against is doing the same type of activity repetitively. Sometimes bodybuilders only do weightlifting, some runners will only run, and some people focusing only on cardiovascular activity will only do cardio classes at the gym. It's important we create different types of fitness for ourselves. Mix it up!

Most of us need to activate our cardiovascular power. Our lives are too sedentary, and we're not moving our bodies the way they're designed to be moving. If you don't use it, you'll lose it. We also need to be adding lean muscle tissue to the body. This can be achieved a lot of different ways and doesn't require hours every day at the gym.

We want to be doing weight-bearing exercises, but you don't need weights. You can do body weight exercises, using your own body weight to achieve muscle development. You can also use dumbbells, free weights, straps, medicine balls, and pulleys at the gym. Machines can help guide your body through the normal ranges of motion they are designed to support. Once you master the machines, move on to free weights for a different kind of challenge that will give you the most natural movement.

Fitness is a necessary component of health, but it's okay to proceed at your own pace. I have noticed not everyone is ready to activate this part of their lifestyle when they are first beginning on a healthier path. If you're not sleeping well and your energy is low, it might not be the best time to exercise. You may need to build your body up first to increase your energy and allow for some healing and better sleep so that your body can handle increasing your fitness level.

When you are exercising, the body is breaking down in order to build up and heal at a stronger level. Not everybody is ready to do that. You always want to listen to your body and acknowledge where you are at that time. However, the moment that you're ready, you should initiate building some lean muscle tissue. In the meantime, gentle exercise such as stretching, swimming, and walking can be started.

The reason why building lean muscle tissue is so important is that, once you hit age thirty-five, you will start losing muscle. You need to continue to rebuild this type of tissue in your body because one day, if you keep losing muscle, you won't be able to help yourself out of a chair. Lean muscle also helps us achieve the physique most of us want.

Building lean muscle tissue has so many health benefits. One of the greatest benefits is an increased metabolism. Lean muscle also helps boost your hormone production, your brain function, and your immune system. It's critical to longevity and to your quality of life as you go through the natural aging process.

Just like I would recommend finding a mentor to guide you through your healing process, I also suggest hiring a personal trainer. If you aren't getting into fitness and enjoying it, if you've had injuries you think are limiting you, or you simply just don't know you're doing, hire a fitness coach to train you.

When you get bored, rather than skipping out, invest in this area to make sure you are continuing on this path. Try a new class. Try a new type of workout. There are a lot of things you can do at home. You don't have to be in a gym. It's good to use a lot of variation when it comes to fitness. Don't just focus on one area. Vary your workouts to combat boredom and plateaus.

Flexibility

Remember my spaghetti example early on in this book?

It applies to our nervous system and to our physical body as well. If you have ever seen a piece of spaghetti that has not been cooked yet, then you know it is dry and brittle, and you can snap it in half. However, if you cook that same piece of spaghetti, and it becomes hydrated and flexible, you can throw it against the wall. It will not break or come apart unless you bite it or cut it. It is much stronger when it is flexible.

Your body is the same way. You need to develop flexibility as well as strength and muscle tone. Your body can handle injuries and daily wear and tear much better when you are more flexible.

Whatever exercise you're doing, be sure you stretch properly. I am a big fan of activities like yoga because they focus on stretching and flexibility, as well as strength. Personally, I like hot yoga because it gives me more of a mental challenge and a deeper stretch. I really notice the difference in my body when I miss my weekly class. Regular un-heated yoga is awesome too. There are many different types of yoga such as vinyasa, yin, hatha, and aerial. Whatever your personality, there is bound to be one that you enjoy.

You can get in the pool where you will have the opportunity to stretch a little bit deeper. Some people like to go in a sauna. An infrared sauna can be a great place to do some stretching and moving. Roll your arms; roll your shoulders around. You don't need a fitness class in order to improve flexibility.

Before and after any regular workouts, you want to make sure you stretch well. Stretching during the day is also beneficial. If you sit at a desk all day, set an alarm on your phone to remind you to periodically walk around and do some stretches. Sitting in the same position for long periods is not healthy. If you are doing repetitive activity throughout your day, take breaks for some different movement and stretching. Actively work on maintaining a healthy flexibility.

Drink a lot of water. Make sure to stay hydrated so your joints are lubricated, and the discs in your spine are hydrated and don't become dried out. Flexibility is not just about stretching but also making sure your hydration and nutrition are up to par. Aim for drinking half your body weight in ounces daily.

It's a simple formula: your weight ÷ 2 = ounces of water per day.

Fun

Exercise should not be something that makes you miserable. While you're moving your body, developing fitness, and increasing flexibility, you want to try to have fun. For me and for many other people, dance is a great way to have fun while exercising. We know that dance increases your feel-good hormones and allows for some good sweating. You can be in your own house, dancing with headphones on. You could go out dancing with your partner or your friends. You could take a class that involves dance. Dance is amazing because you move your body in every single plane; it's not uni-directional like walking, running, or using a cardio machine at the gym.

If you dread going to the gym, that might not be the ideal environment for you. You might need to be creative. Maybe you do better at home. Maybe you do better in a private environment where you are working one-on-one with somebody. Maybe you like classes. Maybe you are an outdoorsy person, so you might like to hike to be out in the fresh air.

Everybody is different. You need to tap into what makes you happy and what allows you to feel the best. Make sure whatever you choose as your activity is fun for you. The more fun you can put into this, the more you are going to get out of it.

STILLNESS

Because we have such busy lives, and there are so many stresses—physical, chemical, and emotional—we are constantly dealing with, it's critical that we stop and take some time to turn inward and quiet our minds as best we can. In these busy times, you need to quiet down and use the power of your mind, the power of calmness and stillness, to create your world, to reset any negativity, and know that you are in control of your day.

Finding time to create some stillness is a key to any successful person's life. Whether you want to be successful in health, business, fitness, or anything else, take the time to quiet down, be grateful, and do some positive, calming techniques to manifest all that you want in your life.

Meditation

Meditation has varied connotations for people. Some love it; they love being calm and going inward. When you say the word *meditate* to other people, however, they may cringe because the last thing they want to do is stop, slow down, and focus inward. Some are so wired they can't calm themselves or their minds. In order to heal, however, they must!

We know that meditation can actually change your brain. There has been research over the years that this type of practice has many neurological benefits. Meditation can change the way your brain is working. It can change your mood and how you participate in your day. Just focusing during this quiet time and allowing yourself the time to meditate can improve concentration and intention. It can reduce anxiety and can help with addiction, anxiety, and depression.

For me, it is a matter of sitting down and having a healthy discipline in my life. When I follow through with this discipline, I am set up for my day. It gives me an opportunity to quiet down and remind myself to be grateful, to focus in on some goals I might have, or the way I want to see things. I use my meditative time as a positive force in creating my best day.

I love going in my infrared sauna and meditating in there. I use chromotherapy in conjunction with a guided chakra meditation, which makes the experience more tangible for me. As a plus, there are no disturbances in the sauna, just peace and alone time, which I know I need. We all need that kind of time.

There are different ways to meditate. You can do transcendental meditation and use the Sanskrit mantra, where you are focusing on that mantra. Other techniques use breathing as a way to meditate. You might focus on doing abdominal breathing exercises, concentrating on the breath, and counting a certain number of seconds in and out. Other forms of meditation are guided, where somebody is talking you through a visual and sensory experience that your brain thinks is actually happening. That can be relaxing and rewarding as well. There are many apps, websites, and resources to help you get started with meditation.

You can begin with a simple five-minute exercise like this:

> Sit down and think of a word that resonates with you and repeat that word over and over. You can use om or so-hum, Sanskrit terms you can look up online to determine if their meaning resonates

with you. You could use a simple visualization instead, like thinking about a color you love or makes you feel peaceful. You need to learn to divert your attention to the present moment so that if you do hear a noise while you are meditating, it becomes a part of your meditation rather than a distraction.

Everybody has thoughts when they meditate. We are all human. Thoughts will come to mind. However, if you can recognize the thought is coming, you can learn to keep yourself from getting caught up in the thought, and instead, allow it to float out of you like a cloud passing by—rather than letting a rainstorm fall on you from that cloud. When you learn to be in control of those thoughts, you will have a much more effective meditation experience.

Breathing

Abdominal breathing is a form of meditation that uses deep breathing to stimulate the relaxation response, to release overall tension, and to create a better sense of well-being. Rather than breathing in a way that is stressed, where your shoulders come up and you are only using your upper body, you want to concentrate on using your whole abdomen and your diaphragm to bring the breath in and push your belly out.

Use abdominal breathing at least twice a day and any time you find yourself in a stressful situation or having negative thoughts. It should only take a few minutes. Use it if you are having pain. Often, when we experience these difficulties, our breathing becomes shallow and abdominal breathing can help.

You can train yourself to do abdominal breathing:

> First, start with one hand on your chest and the other on your abdomen. When you take a deep breath in, you should feel the hand on your stomach rising higher than the one on your chest. You could be sitting or lying down for this. Take a deep breath in through your nose and hold it for a count of seven. You could also take the breath while you are counting; take a slow breath in for seven seconds, and then let the breath out on the count of eight.
>
> Counting and focusing on the breath is a form of meditation. Activate your abdominal muscles to push the majority of the air from your lungs as you are exhaling. Take a breath in through your nose and push the breath out, repeating this at least five times.
>
> If you like, you can do some positive affirmations now:
>
> *I am so grateful I got a bonus today at work.*
>
> *I got an A on my test.*

I hit my goal with my health.

I had a great night's sleep.

I am so happy and grateful that I am an amazing person, and I make a difference in the world.

I am a great mom.

Add whatever your goals are and continue with the breathing to enhance your experience. I find appreciation to be very meaningful and it keeps me in a positive mindset. Bad day? Focus on what you're grateful for!

Once you feel comfortable with this, you won't need to put your hands on your body because you will naturally know what it should feel like. This is a good starting point for additional meditation practices. Practice thinking positive thoughts. Focus on anything that can relax your mind. You may like to picture yourself somewhere relaxing, like at the beach, while you are doing breathing exercises.

When you find yourself in a stressful situation, you can use meditation to help manage your stress. Stop and take a couple of minutes to do these breathing exercises. Stress is at the root of all our ills. In order to address our health for the long term, we have to address the stresses that are the causes.

Using Your Thoughts to Create Your Life

Most people have heard of the law of attraction. When we call something a law, this means it works every time. For example, the law of gravity tells us if I take a pen and hold it up, every time I let go of it, it will fall to the ground. It is a law.

When people think about the law of attraction, they might think that this means when they wish for something, it will magically show up in their life. It doesn't really happen exactly that way. Yes, we need to think about those things happening, but we need to think about them *as if they have already happened and we truly believe.*

For example, if you have a goal of losing twenty pounds, part of the process should be thinking: *I am so happy and grateful that I lost twenty pounds, and I am sleeping fantastically. I am full of energy. I feel ten years younger.* You think about your goal as if it has already happened, or is happening in that moment.

According to Earl Nightengale in *the Strangest Secret* (Dead Authors Society, 2018), you want to set a definite date for the manifestation of your goal to happen. The teachings of Abraham Hicks, on the other hand, say it's already happening as you believe and raise your vibration to match the feeling of achieving the goal, even though the time is not something we can choose. If it's a vibrational match and we are allowing, then you will receive that which you desire. This suggests that the choosing a definite time is not necessary, and manifestations happen quickly if you are in alignment.

Proclaiming what you want to the universe helps it manifest—so write it down, say it out loud, and attach emotion to it. Write down how achieving that goal will help you and how you will feel when you're there. Then take action. Create your life.

Thinking must be intentional. When you have negative thoughts, you are going to add more negativity in your life. You are sending out a vibrational frequency to match that negativity. When you have positive thoughts, you are going to get more positivity in your life. Catch yourself when you are being negative or when you are not having a healthy response to a situation. You can stop yourself and change. Most of us naturally go to negativity. That is how we have been trained in this world we live in. It only takes a few extra seconds to stop yourself and turn it into something positive. You must deliberately work on this until it becomes more natural.

For example, when someone cuts you off on the road, it is easy to get annoyed or maybe even want to yell at them from inside your car. I am the first one to do this. But maybe something happened to a member of that person's family; maybe they are in a hurry and aren't thinking. Maybe someone needs their help, and they are in a rush to get there. We don't know what is going on in someone else's life.

You might automatically have a negative response, but you can stop yourself. Maybe you can say: *I send them love and light. Whatever is going on, I hope they will be safe, and everything will be okay.* You can lead yourself in a more peaceful state that way.

To create your life, thoughts must come first and then action. You must ask the universe for something. The universe is already lining this up for you. It is your job to create the space for it to happen. Things don't just magically show up in our lives. We need to change our thoughts and move into alignment.

Thoughts are the first part of the work. Actions are next.

The law of attraction has the word action in it, doesn't it?

Don't worry about the *how*, that part is not really what I am talking about. The *how* will show up when you are in alignment. It's more the *why* that will help you get there.

You must take action if you really want to see your dreams come into fruition the way you have designed them. You are in control. When it comes to your health, you must create these thoughts, visions, and goals for yourself. They will manifest when you are in a calmer state. Using the creative thought process along with meditation and breathing will allow you to achieve your dreams at a much faster pace.

AWARENESS

You are the only you.

According to Dr. Ali Benazir's article on the probability of being born, Dr. Binazir says, "The probability of being you is about one in four hundred trillion. You are a miracle. You are an unlikely event, practically impossible for you to even happen."[16]

I want you to have the best health and life possible. Taking steps each day will ensure that. Creating self-awareness is the true path to healing. Self-awareness is the conscious knowledge of one's own character, feelings, motives, and desires.

What does this mean when it comes to your health?

You want to make sure that you are developing self-awareness. Tune in and connect with your body not just in pleasure but also in pain. There is meaning in everything we experience. Be conscious of your mindset; some people don't even realize they are in a negative mindset all the time.

Explore your own patterns of thought:

- *How do I think?*
- *What do I find meaningful?*

16 Binazir, Ali. "Are you a Miracle? On the Probability of Your Being Born." *Huffpost.* 16 June 2011. https://www.huffpost.com/entry/probability-being-born_b_877853

- *What am I passionate about?*
- *What are my interests?*
- *What do I love?*
- *What are my beliefs, both empowering and limiting?*
- *What are my values?*
- *What was I put here on Earth to do?*
- *What emotions do I feel most of the time?*

If you are feeling anger most of the time, this is something you need to address. There is something underneath creating that.

Ask yourself: *What am I feeling right now? What are my needs right now?*

Some people feel like they need to go to the refrigerator, but what they really need is a hug or some physical touch or someone to tell them they love them. We must learn to tune in to what our body is really telling us. This is such a huge advantage when it comes to everything in life.

Listening to Your Body

Your body will tell you what you need to know if you just listen.

Have you ever had a gut instinct about something, where you could just feel in the pit of your stomach that something wasn't right?

Your body was telling you something wasn't right. Maybe you listened, or maybe you ignored it. In my life, any time I have ignored the gut instinct, it has come back to bite me. Any time I have listened, tuned in, and followed my gut instincts, it has paid off in dividends.

Listen to your body. Messages can come in many different ways. Maybe it is not just gut instinct.

Suppose you stub your toe. Ask yourself: *What am I being told by that stubbed toe?* You're being told pay attention. You're not in the present moment.

Suppose you're having headaches and have been popping Tylenol all day to deal with them. You're not listening to your body; you're masking what your body is telling you instead of addressing WHY you are having headaches.

Suppose you're having a chronic pain that won't go away no matter what you do. According to Louise Hay, different parts of the body experiencing different symptoms are indications of things in your life that are manifesting physically.

Look at your body and listen to it. If you can find connections there, think about what they mean in your life. You will be more in control of your body and health and your life in general. You will be more in control of the experiences that you are having here, whether they be positive or negative.

Self-awareness is the true path to healing. When you listen to your body, it will tell you what you need.

When it comes to diet, if you are eating the same foods all the time, you probably won't notice if those foods are making you sick. When you stop eating those foods for a while and then reintroduce them, your body will tell you what the right foods are for you.

I recently had a practice member, Robert, who used to eat eggs all the time. I had him stop eating eggs for six weeks. Some time later, he had a hardboiled egg and he couldn't even believe how sick he got. Now he is totally averse to eggs. He doesn't want to eat them because he knows they are inflammatory for him. That same man has just about reversed his diabetes through the very methods I have taught you in this book. It just gives you an idea of what we can do when we really tune in and listen.

Our body is an incredible messenger, if we would only listen.

A Calm Nervous System

You have the best doctor in the world residing right inside of you. You were born with it. It is called your innate intelligence. Your innate intelligence has a laundry list of importance. You are an incredible healing machine! Trust your body. Don't be afraid of symptoms; know that your body is not to be feared but is a messenger for you. It will heal what is more life endangering first. People become disappointed when the very thing they want to heal is last on that list. Be patient with your healing process. There may be a missing piece, but your innate intelligence may just be checking off the list one by one.

We all know the brain is a master computer. It controls all the other systems in the body. Many of us don't realize that we are in a constant state of fight-or-flight because of all the stresses in our lives. This fight-or-flight response is not supposed to be present all the time. It was a helpful response for our ancestors if there was a tiger nearby, and they had to either run or fight. In this busy world, because we are constantly bombarded by physical, chemical, and emotional stress, our bodies get stuck in this state of fight-or-flight.

When we are in a state of fight-or-flight, the blood goes to the extremities. When the blood is in the extremities, this means it is not in the vital organs working to help our bodies function at an optimal level. We do not sleep well, digest well, or heal well, and it wipes out our libido.

When we are in the midst of this stress response, we have increased adrenaline that boosts our energy. There is a purpose to it if you need to run; increased blood pressure moves more oxygen to your muscles, which increases your pulse; increased muscle tension enables you to be able to take action; dilated pupils enable you to see better. However, your digestive process, your immune system, and your sexual functions slow down because these are not necessary in a fight-or-flight situation.

We need to move ourselves out of this fight-or-flight state into a calmer state so our bodies can function better, absorb nutrients better, digest better, and sleep better. This is how we are going to be able to heal.

We need to maintain a calm nervous system if we want all these other body systems to be effective, and we want our brain and body to have great communication. Your nerves and spinal cord are responsible for communication from the brain to the body and vice versa, and you don't want to have any static on your line. You don't want any interference in your nervous system. You want to have healthy communication from the body to the brain and the brain to the body.

Having that calm nervous system will allow everything else you're doing to be more effective. We can achieve this using all the ways mentioned above. I also recommend receiving regular chiropractic care. It was Network Spinal Analysis (NSA) that really started me on my healing journey, and I will never negate the impact that had on my potential for healing. I do believe having a healthy connection between the body and brain and releasing tension on my nervous system allowed for the changes needed for me to heal. That made a huge difference for me.

We also want to be measuring how well our nervous system is handling stress. I use heart rate variability (HRV) testing in the office as a measuring tool. Heart Math™ has a free app that goes along with an earpiece you connect to your smartphone, so you can work on your stress levels on your own. It is a great tool, a very under-utilized tool. HRV feedback using Heart Math puts you in the driver's seat. The more we realize we can be in control of our health, the more empowered we will be to have our health and wellness in the long term. Line up your mind, thoughts, and emotions to Awaken Wellness.

Question Everything

I always tell people to question everything because it was questioning everything that brought me where I am today. Before I found this lifestyle—where I am in control of my health, I am in control of my emotions, my thoughts, and ultimately, I am in charge of my life as a result—I just followed what I was told. I was told to go to the doctor when I had a symptom. I was told to get a flu shot. I was told to be quiet, not question anything, and just follow along with what everyone else was doing.

A very long time ago, a brilliant man named Bob Proctor once said something along the lines of, "Chances are, if you are following the crowd, you're on the wrong path."

Adopting this as my truth has put me in the most empowered and inspired position I could possibly be in. That is what I wish for everyone to have. To have this awareness. To be awake.

There are powers at large that don't want you to know everything, that don't want you to question everything. This isn't about conspiracy theories. It's about law and order and controlling the population in certain ways. It's okay for us to branch off, to realize we don't have to follow. We don't have to be part of the herd of cows.

My friend, Laura, who was helping me tap into my inner soul energy, said to me, "You're like a fish swimming in a school with millions of other fish. You just decide, 'Screw this,' and 'I'm going the other way.' You go the other way, but everyone is bumping into you. They're knocking you over. You keep getting back up and keep going."

That is what it is like when you turn against what most people are doing. Just because something is common doesn't mean it's normal.

I encourage you to question everything, including me, and find your own path. Recognize you are your own person with your own thoughts and feelings, your own health, your own experience, your own relationships, your own history, your own traumas, and your own happiness.

Come into who you are as an individual, to be the happiest person you can be, to live your purpose to the fullest, and to make this life the best life that you can. That is what it's all about.

I am so grateful I have found Dr. Nicole. She really understands health in a way that is so unique to find in any doctor. She is passionate and on a mission to bring healing, or even better, help people find their own healing. From the moment I saw her website online when "shopping around" for a functional medicine doctor, my gut told me this was the right place. But then I never called. It was months later when something within me spoke to me to make that call and go for it. Since I took that leap at the end of August 2018, my life has been changed in so many immeasurable ways. I knew the moment I walked in the doors of her office and I felt at home I was in the right place and I was in good hands. I have complex health issues that my conventional medical doctors would never have gotten to the bottom of. My wellness journey would not be complete without Dr. Nicole, and I am glad to be on this path with her. I am also grateful for her help with my husband and feel very ready to entrust her to help my three kids do the same. If you are browsing and not sure if you should call or sign up with Dr. Nicole, don't hesitate!! Please do it!!!!

~ Amy Krostich

Conclusion

I realize I've given you a lot of information in this very short book. Believe it or not, there is still a lot more to learn.

There is so much confusion today about what to do to heal our bodies. The level of knowledge required to be totally awakened and aware is massive, and we have barely scratched the surface. It is my hope that this book helps you begin to make more conscious decisions every day to create better health for you and for your family. Just try to make changes one step at a time, and over time you will take control back of your health and life.

We are all different, so when it comes to healing our own unique challenges, most people need help. It is often difficult to decipher for yourself what is going on inside your body, and it is hard to motivate yourself and keep yourself accountable. It's also hard to know the proper steps you need to take and in what order to take them. That is why having a mentor and guide to coach and inspire you through this process makes a huge difference.

If you would like my help in this process, I would be very happy to help you, no matter where you live. I am able to help people anywhere. You can visit my website at www. DrNicole.com for more information on how you can take the next steps.

You may be an athlete wanting to optimize your performance; you may be dealing with a major diagnosis such as diabetes or an autoimmune disease; you may even be facing surgery at this point. I do not treat any of these conditions, but I can help you heal your own body and become self-reliant in maintaining your health and wellness.

The way to achieve this is by concentrating on the five pillars of health: proper detoxification, healing nutrition, purposeful movement, natural hormone balancing, and a calm, clear nervous system that handles stress well. Pair these pillars with mentoring and a solid wellness education, and you will be empowered and independent, not just to get your health back, but to keep it. Awaken Wellness!

It is never too late to look for the cause of your problems instead of merely treating symptoms. Don't give up!

You want to keep in mind that there is no destination; health is a lifetime journey. Of course, there are specific goals you would like to achieve, but learning the tools for longevity and how to care for your ongoing health is key.

Remember, we want to make sure we are healing our bodies on all levels, not just physical. We have emotional, chemical, spiritual, intellectual, and mental needs. There are many aspects of us we need to get in alignment for us to have not just the best health, but also the best life. Maintaining health will extend your life, but it will also improve the quality of your life. Your best quality of life will enable you to live your purpose and to have the best relationships you can with loved ones and with yourself.

It's about doing all the things you want to do. Maybe your dreams are to travel, to have a successful business, or to be the best mom. You just can't do what you want when you don't feel good. Your health, good or bad, impacts your entire life.

Health is your greatest asset. Invest in it. If you don't, you will have a debt to pay at some point. It's never too late. If you have neglected your health for a long time, you may have some bigger challenges, but there are always steps you can take to work toward the betterment of your health and your life. If there is breath, there is hope.

It is my sincere hope that this book has left you empowered and encouraged to take action. Get in touch with me at drnicole@drnicole.com and take that very first step toward the realization of your health goals. I'm here to mentor you through the process and give you customized, individualized advice specific to your situation and your needs. I look forward to hearing from you soon.

In closing, I leave you with this proverb:

> *When you have your health,*
> *you have a thousand dreams;*
> *when you don't, you only have one.*

Next Steps

If you are looking for an experienced mentor to help you on your path back to health, regardless of your condition, please call me at 561-740-2340. I am also available for speaking engagements or keynote speeches.

For more information, you can visit my website at www. DrNicole.com.

Please contact me at DrNicole@DrNicole.com, and I will be happy to set up a complimentary fifteen-minute phone consultation so we can get acquainted and explore what we can do to help you move forward on your health journey to reach your health goals. If you are local, I would love to have you join me at one of my seminars. If you aren't local, it's okay, I can still work with you wherever you are.

In order to provide natural healthcare, education, healthy food, and clean water to the underserved in our world and locally, I started a chapter of Hands for Life. To make a donation to Hands for Life, go to www.HandsforLifeEBB.org

About the Author

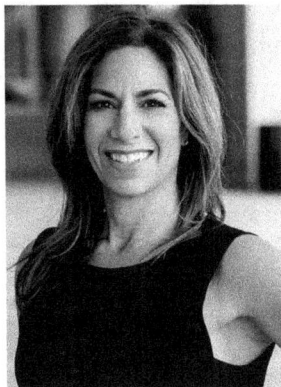

Dr. Nicole Rothman is a Doctor of Chiropractic with a post-graduate focus on functional wellness and functional nutrition, along with lifestyle wellness. Some call this type of practice *functional medicine*. She also received her two-hundred-hour certification from Academy Council of Chiropractic Pediatrics in 2016. She attended Life College of Chiropractic, graduating in 1997, and received her doctorate. She received her bachelor of science in biology in 1993 from the University of Albany. In 1998, Dr. Rothman opened her practice in Boynton Beach, where she has helped thousands of people, adults and children, reclaim their health and lives through her *Awaken Wellness* programs.

In 2017, she created the *Awakened Wellness Blueprint* to help clients reclaim health, youth, and life, where she incorporates the five pillars of health within her curriculum and combines it with program customization and mentoring in order to help people achieve optimal results. She motivates them to control not just their health, but to be in control of their lives. Dr. Rothman has been attending life-transformational workshops and seminars since the mid-90s. She has been to Inner Winners, The Gathering, Tony Robbins, and many more. She has challenged herself to walk on fire, bend six-foot steel reinforcement bars with her throat, break boards, and more.

Dr. Rothman has been involved in charitable efforts in her community for over twenty years. She has hosted many fundraising events, including school-supply drives, backpack drives, and pajama drives, and recently launched the Hands for Life East Boynton Beach chapter in her community to allow the underserved to access her *Awakened Wellness* program. She served on an overseas chiropractic mission in 1997, which encouraged her to intensify her efforts back here at home in America, realizing the people of our country need just as much help as they do abroad.

She loves to travel the world and especially enjoys quality time creating memories with her husband, Troy, her two adult children, Elijah and Levi, and her cockapoo, GG. Her passion is to inspire others to recognize their human potential. This is evident in her daily life. She walks the talk, and how she lives is what she teaches to others. Her greatest joy is helping someone take control of their health and heal themselves.